Administrative and Clinical Procedures for the Health Office Professional

VALERIE D. THOMPSON

CONESTOGA COLLEGE OF APPLIED ARTS AND TECHNOLOGY

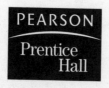

PEARSON

Prentice Hall

Toronto

National Library of Canada Cataloguing in Publication

Thompson, Valerie D., 1948–
    Administrative and clinical procedures for the health
office professional / Valerie D. Thompson.

Includes index.
ISBN 0-13-076560-0

    1. Medical offices—Management. 2. Medical assistants.
3. Physicians' assistants. I. Title.

R728.8.T53 2005   651'.961   C2004-901615-6

ISBN 0-13-076560-0

Vice President, Editorial Director: Michael J. Young
Executive Acquisitions Editor: Samantha Scully
Executive Marketing Manager: Cas Shields
Developmental Editor: Paul Donnelly
Production Editor: Joel Gladstone
Copy Editor: Rohini Herbert
Substantive Editor: Gilda Mekler
Production Coordinator: Andrea Falkenberg
Page Layout: Debbie Kumpf, Christine Velakis
Art Director: Mary Opper
Interior and cover design: Lisa LaPointe
Cover Image: Photodisc
Illustrations: Jillian Pinder

6 WC 09 08

Visual Practice Software Images supplied courtesy of Advanced Computer Systems Limited. Copyright © 2004. All rights expressly reserved. http://www.visualpractice.com

Statistics Canada information is used with permission of the Minister of Industry, as Minister responsible for Statistics Canada. Information on the availability of the wide range of data from Statistics Canada can be obtained from Statistics Canada's Regional Offices, its World Wide Web site at www.statcan.ca, and its toll-free access number 1-800-263-1136.

Printed and bound in Canada.

To my husband, Doug, whose patience, support and expert medical advice have been invaluable. To Spencer, Leigh, Stephanie, Chad, and Regan, for understanding my need to remain 'focused' over the past two years, and for their support. To administrative staff in all sectors of health care who provide such an essential service for clients and health practitioners alike.

Brief Contents

Contents

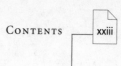

Historical Overview

The Health Office: The Medical Secretary

The role of the health office professional has shifted over the years, becoming more responsible and complex (see Figure 1.1).

Administrative assistants were introduced to health care in the early 1920s. Prior to that, physicians assumed nearly all administrative and clinical responsibilities in their practices. If they needed help, they recruited a spouse, family member, or friend. Formal training was neither considered nor readily available. Early doctor's assistants performed

---

1955

Busy medical office requires secretary. Needs good telephone skills. Good with people. Will train. Start immediately.

1965

Busy doctor's office requires medical secretary to start immediately. Commercial course required. Typing skills, good with people, organized. Knowledge of medical terminology an asset. Duties include booking appointments, answering the telephone, billing, general office duties.

1970

Medical Secretary urgently sought by Cardiologist. Successful candidate must have secretarial training: typing, dicta typing, medical terminology, bookkeeping skills required. Previous experience an asset. Duties include filing, billing, telephone management, processing mail, and maintaining inventory. Salary commensurate with experience.

1980

Medical Secretary required by group practice. Certificate in related program an asset. Must know medical terminology, medical transcription, typing, and accounts receivable/payroll. Good telephone and communication skills. Pleasant manner. Duties include general office management, provincial billing, maintaining medical records, and referrals. Apply with resume to Dr. M. Black, 222 Brunswick Street, Burnaby.

1990

Medical secretary for busy solo practice. Graduate of a health administration course an asset. Excellent communication skills a must. Previous experience an asset. Duties include booking appointments, provincial billing, medical transcription. Health care terminology a must. Must be a team player, multitasker, organized, with a pleasant, outgoing personality. Apply with resume to Dr. R. Collins. 111 Chester Ave., Sheffield. Ph 233-2222

2004

Full-time medical secretary/office administrator required for busy solo OB/GYN office. Individual must have a dynamic personality and possess good interpersonal communication and interviewing skills. Must work well under stress and be able to multitask. Graduate of a 2 year health office administration program from a community college or equivalent. Experience with Microsoft Word and Excel mandatory. Familiarity with medical software an asset. Duties include provincial billing, error-free dictatyping, taking vital signs, appointment and OR scheduling, triage. Must work well as a team member. Reconciliation experience a plus. Fax resume to 111-2222.

Figure 1.1   Advertisements for a medical secretary as they would have appeared over the last 50 years show the growing complexity and breadth of skills required from the 1950s to today.

varied tasks, and their role was often not clearly defined. Appointment schedules were maintained informally, if at all. Clients were seen randomly instead of by appointment, and physicians commonly made house calls instead of seeing clients in the office. Client records, filing systems, and billing procedures were informal or nonexistent. Often, reimbursement was a direct exchange between physician and client. Sometimes, payment involved barter, with clients paying in produce or whatever they had to give. Patients paid what they could, when they could. Seldom did the physician force the issue if a client was unable to pay. There was no insurance, and often there was no record of payment. The client's medical history, for the most part, was what the client, the physician, and his assistant (if any) could remember.

As medical knowledge and technology advanced, physicians became more focused on their practices and responsibilities in the office, clinic, and the hospital setting. Arrangements between the doctor and the patient became more formalized, and a more clearly defined role emerged for the office assistant. Most doctors began to rely on an assistant with office skills to handle the administrative components of their practice; many also found that they required clinical assistance. Thus, some office assistants or medical secretaries had a purely administrative role, and others took on clinical responsibilities as well.

Academic Change

Components of formal training for office professionals appeared in the mid-20th century. High schools offered commercial or business courses that included bookkeeping or accounting, and typing. Communication skills were also important. Medical secretaries added to these skills with on-the-job training. Later, command of medical terminology and medical **transcription** skills became added requirements, and formal secretarial training became more popular.

TRANSCRIPTION creating a written copy of a dictated or recorded message.

Today, health office professionals must be computer literate and knowledgeable, among other things, about provincial billing, pharmacology, laboratory and diagnostic tests, ethics, and human relations. Many community colleges and independent business colleges offer health administration programs, which vary from a one-year certificate program to a two- or three-year diploma program. Some programs are accelerated, offering, for example, a two-year diploma program in a shorter time frame. Many colleges integrate simulated office experiences or co-op or workplace experience, either throughout the program or at the end.

The Hospital

Hospital nurses were originally responsible for all administrative functions as well as client care. As client care became more complex, nurses more skilled, and demands heavier, the need for administrative assistance became increasingly evident. The position of the **ward clerk** was introduced to take care of such tasks as answering the telephone; informing clients about hospital rules and regulations; preparing, maintaining, and disassembling charts; ordering supplies; handing out and collecting diet sheets; graphing vital signs on the client's chart; posting notices and schedules; and updating admissions and discharge lists.

WARD CLERK an individual who manages the administrative and communication needs of a client care unit. The title is being replaced with "clinical secretary" and "communications coordinator."

The ward clerk was not allowed to process doctors' orders, take laboratory or diagnostic reports over the telephone, or respond to most physician requests. These tasks were primarily the responsibility of the head nurse. In the past few years, the term *ward clerk* has been replaced in many settings by *clinical secretary, clerical associate,* or *communications coordinator* to better reflect increased responsibilities, notably, transcribing physicians' orders. The clinical secretary coordinates written and oral communication and plays key administrative roles. These positions are usually filled by health office administration graduates or by long-standing employees who have gained a wealth of knowledge on the job. The duties and responsibilities of the clinical secretary are discussed in more detail in Chapter 15.

Employment Opportunities

Positions

Health office professionals work in a wide variety of positions with different titles and duties. The following summary outlines some of the more common ones.

Medical Office Assistant

The role of **medical assistant** is more clearly defined in the United States than in Canada. In the United States, the medical assistant primarily assists the physician with clinical tasks but may also handle some administrative responsibilities. This term is often used in British Columbia as well. In most of Canada, however, the more common term is **medical office assistant**, and this job description generally includes more administrative than clinical responsibilities. Medical assistants in the United States are trained to take blood specimens, administer injections, give oral medications, administer electrocardiograms and other laboratory tests, and perform other specialized tasks—tasks generally performed by nurses in Canada. Medical assistants also take vital signs, prepare patients for procedures, take histories, prepare the examination or treatment room, assess client need when scheduling appointments, and determine when patients need to be seen urgently. Canadian health office professionals assume many of these responsibilities in some health-care settings.

> **MEDICAL ASSISTANT** (U.S.) a person who is trained to assist a physician with various clinical tests, examinations, and procedures.
>
> **MEDICAL OFFICE ASSISTANT** (Canada) a person who handles primarily administrative but also some clinical duties in a health office.

Integrating some nursing duties into the health office professional's job is not new but is becoming more common as the changing face of health care demands multiskilled, versatile, and cost-effective workers. In some offices, the health office professional assumes expanded duties such as giving allergy shots and assisting with procedures. The health office professional must be trained by the doctor to carry out these tasks, some of which are legally considered "delegated acts," meaning that the physician takes responsibility for the employee's actions.

Administrative Nursing Coordinator

An increasing number of community agencies supply a range of in-home medical services, especially home-based nursing care to clients discharged from hospital with conditions requiring ongoing care and assessment. Community nurses start and maintain intravenous (IV) therapy in the home, apply dressings, and maintain clients on respirators. These clients may have chest tubes and other complex medical interventions. Clients are routinely admitted to the agencies' services and discharged when their need for care terminates. Each agency needs someone in an administrative role, often called a *nursing coordinator,* to coordinate the agency's needs and activities. This person is aware of the caseloads of various nurses, assigns new admissions on the basis of caseload and priority, conveys vital information about clients' medical needs, and keeps track of admissions and discharges. To take on this role, you must be aware of the responsibilities of the various types of nurses within the organization and the related scope of practice for each group (discussed in detail in Chapter 15). You must be able to prioritize information and be familiar with medications, critical lab values, and other components of community care.

Medical Transcriptionist

A medical transcriptionist produces medical reports, correspondence, records, client-care information, statistics, medical research, and administrative material. In a hospital, transcriptionists are members of a larger team in the Medical Records, or Information Health, Department. The transcriptionist listens to recorded reports or reads rough notes and produces formal reports in document form. In highly computerized environments, the transcriptionist edits and formats documents that have been transcribed by voice-activated technology. Documents transcribed include discharge summaries, referral letters, and reports on histories, physical examinations, operations, consultations, autopsies, radiology examinations, and obstetrics.

As well as specific training in transcription, the medical transcriptionist must have general medical knowledge, sound judgment, and logical and problem-solving abilities. A good transcriptionist can spot mistakes in a report and check when neccessary with the doctor to get the right information.

Occupational Settings

A wide variety of positions are available for the health office professional. The health-care field is diverse, and opportunities continue to broaden as the industry restructures and the roles of health-care professionals change. Occupational settings range from the fast-paced challenge of the emergency room to the less hectic environment of a specialist's office, and from a busy walk-in clinic with a lot of client contact to a Medical Records Department with limited public contact.

Many positions are also available in sectors of the allied health-care and alternative health-care fields. The health office professional is considered to be part of the allied health-care field, along with other professions more centred on direct client care. **Allied health care** includes any duty or function that supports primary health-care professionals, such as physicians, in the delivery of health-care services. Allied health-care professions include physiotherapists, osteopaths, midwives, and nurses. Many of these professionals are in independent practice while working collaboratively with other health-care professionals. For example, with the current move to community-based care, there has been an increase in the number of independent nursing service organizations. Some sectors of the allied health-care industry offer valuable employment opportunities for the health office professional.

Alternative health care, also referred to as **complementary health care**, is considered by most to be the natural approach to treating the causes of illness and disease. Alternative health care includes nontraditional methods and practices, such as chiropractic, acupuncture, massage, and aromatherapy. These professions offer the consumer a replacement or an adjunct to traditional health care. Alternative health-care professions are growing in number and popularity.

Many allied, alternative, and mainstream health-care professionals work independently and/or in facilities that offer the client collaborative care, as well as a range of health-care choices. Alternative and allied health-care professionals provide employment opportunities for the health office professional with duties and responsibilities similar to those in traditional health-care offices. Throughout this book, we focus primarily on physicians' offices and hospitals, the two settings most covered in health administration courses, as it would be impossible to do justice to the whole range of possibilities in a single textbook. But keep in mind that your basic skills and knowledge can take you in many directions.

You might find a job in any of the following workplaces—and even this list is not complete.

ALLIED HEALTH CARE any duty or profession that supports primary health-care professionals, such as physicians, in delivering health-care services.

ALTERNATIVE HEALTH CARE or COMPLEMENTARY HEALTH CARE nontraditional methods and practices, based on a natural approach, including chiropractic, acupuncture, massage, and aromatherapy.

Office and Community

- Doctor's office (group or solo practice), generalist or specialist
- Ambulatory care or walk-in clinic (also may be called an urgent care clinic)
- Dental offices
- Optometry offices
- Nurse practitioner's office
- Community agencies, such as Public Health
- Victorian Order of Nurses (VON)
- Canadian Red Cross
- Canadian Cancer Society
- CCAC (Community Care Access Centre) or equivalent
- Independent community health-care agencies

Clinics (often connected with hospitals)

- Orthopedics
- Prenatal/postpartum/birthing centres
- Diabetic
- Mental health
- Systemic therapy
- Renal dialysis
- Oncology
- Palliative care
- Laser surgery clinics

Alternative/Allied Health-Care Facilities

- Acupuncture
- Reflexology
- Massage therapy
- Aromatherapy
- Chiropractor
- Osteopath

Hospital Departments

- Admitting/Patient (Client) Registration
- Medical Records/Information Health
- Emergency Room
- Laboratory (various departments within the laboratory)
- Maternal/Child
- Pediatrics
- Medicine
- Surgery
- Operating Room
- Social Services
- Radiology

Health-Care Facilities

- Long-term care facilities (nursing homes)
- Seniors' residences
- Rehabilitative centres

CLINIC a facility providing medical care on an outpatient basis. Many clinics have a specialty, such as ongoing care for diabetes or cancer.

A workplace experience component may also be called a co-op (cooperative experience), practicum (practical application of skills), consolidation (an experience wherein the student consolidates acquired skills and theory), or externship (getting experience outside of the college environment).

The workplace experience involves a contractual agreement among the employer, the student, and the college. The time frame varies with the length and structure of the program. The purpose of this experience is to provide the student with the chance to put theory to practice—to apply the skills learned in college to the workplace setting. The student is able to assume some job responsibilities while still under the guidance of a **preceptor**, or someone whom the student can turn to for guidance and advice.

PRECEPTOR a mentor who guides and supervises a student throughout a workplace experience.

In most co-op programs, students can seek placement in an area of interest, assuming suitable opportunities are available and the experience offered matches program requirements. Most facilities require the student to apply for the experience, in the same manner as one would for a job. Students thus gain experience with résumés and interviews. If more than one student applies for the same opening, the selection should be based on suitability, just as in any job competition. Do not take it personally if you are not selected—and make sure to apply for more than one position. Some programs do not use an application process; instead, the employer asks the program coordinator or a placement officer to select the best-suited student. Usually, student requests are an important part of any decisions made.

Cooperative work experiences offer

- the opportunity to apply what you have learned in college to a practical setting;
- general work experience;
- personal insight into your own abilities, strengths, and needs for improvement; and
- the opportunity to develop a level of professionalism and professional ethics.

Expectations and Responsibilities

The employer has the right to expect that the student involved in the experience is qualified (at an entry level) and will abide by the workplace's rules. In health-care settings, for example, where health office professionals frequently have access to confidential client records, students may be required to sign a confidentiality statement.

The college and the student have the right to expect that the employer will provide an experience that reflects the objectives and expectations outlined by the initial agreement. On occasion, an employer will view the student as merely an extra set of hands, forgetting that the student is there to complete a set of learning outcomes. Students should discuss such problems with their preceptors or employers and, if they remain unresolved, with their faculty advisors.

Student Preparation

Before entering a workplace experience, you must be prepared and organized. To ensure you start off on the right foot, you should meet with the employer and/or preceptor before accepting a position to review your own and the employer's expectations and to determine the duties and responsibilities of the position. Review all relevant materials, such as evaluation criteria, with the appropriate persons. Discuss the evaluation tool itself and how often evaluations will take place. Most health-care facilities require a visible liaison between the facility and the faculty advisor for the duration of the student's experience. Find out what type of contact will occur and how often; if possible, set up appointments in advance. Review your responsibilities to the college to ensure that there are no mix-ups or misunderstandings. Some colleges will expect you to send your faculty advisor weekly summaries or to submit a final paper on completion of the workplace experience.

Evaluation

Evaluations should be done at regular intervals during any cooperative experience—every two weeks is not unreasonable—to provide continuous feedback and allow the student and the employer to discuss any problems as they arise. Positive feedback is equally important. Knowing that you are doing a good job provides you with confidence and a sense of accomplishment. If you feel that you are not getting positive feedback, tactfully ask for it. "What do you see as my strengths during these past two weeks?" "In what areas do you feel I am best suited to this experience?" Self-evaluations are also helpful and should normally resemble the employer's evaluation. If the two are very different, the reasons need to be investigated.

Employment Expectations

Any workplace or co-op experience should be viewed as if it were an actual job. Approach the experience with a positive attitude and a sense of commitment. Act like a professional, in dress, manner, and attitude. Be punctual, and notify the employer if you are ill. Seek out new learning opportunities, complete tasks in a timely manner, demonstrate organizational skills, and try to work harmoniously with other team members. Although it is important to work as independently as possible, it is equally important to recognize your limitations, seek help appropriately, and work within your designated **scope of practice**. Not adhering to this can cause difficulties for you, your preceptor or employer, and perhaps others.

A cooperative experience may lead to employment, but there is no guarantee, and you should not enter into it with that expectation. A positive cooperative experience will, however, provide you with a good reference to add to your résumé.

SCOPE OF PRACTICE
working within the parameters of duties and responsibilities outlined by one's professional training and skill set.

Continuing Education

Graduating from an accredited program as a health-care professional is only the first step in the educational process. Most community colleges and independent educational centres across Canada offer courses in a wide range of clinical and administrative skills. You may be required to take courses to keep abreast of technological and communication advances within the administrative setting or to prepare you to assume a wider range of responsibilities in your current job setting. Many colleges articulate with universities, offering advanced standing to college graduates wanting to pursue a degree in Health Administration. Athabaska University in Alberta is one such facility. The trend to expect multiple skills will continue to grow. Continued learning is not only a professional responsibility—a duty to yourself as well as your employer—but is an effective way to broaden your career opportunities. Employers value self-motivation and the combination of experience and additional educational qualifications. Keeping abreast of the latest administrative procedures and technological advances makes you a valuable asset to any health-care setting.

Summary

1. Health office professionals have many different job titles, depending on the areas in which they work. Advancing technology and the changing Canadian health-care system have created a need for knowledgeable, multiskilled people in administrative positions. Most employers now seek graduates of certificate or diploma programs.

2. Health office professionals find work in many settings, including medical and other health-care offices, specialty clinics, alternative and allied health-care facilities, hospital departments, long-term care facilities, seniors' residences, government offices, and companies. Employment is expected to grow.

3. Desirable attributes of the health office professional include a friendly, approachable personality, a sense of responsibility, flexibility, good judgment, and the ability to remain calm in stressful situations. Although these attributes are inherent, some people have to work to develop them.

4. Professionalism is reflected in dress, thought, speech, and action. As the health office professional is usually the client's first contact, a positive first impression is important. While dress codes vary, cleanliness, neatness, and appropriateness always apply.

5. Skills, while they may overlap with attributes, are generally learned. Communication skills are essential, including clear enunciation, excellent spoken and written grammar, sensitive listening, and the ability to express empathy and to understand and convey information clearly. Keyboarding, computer literacy, and the ability to understand, use, and write medical terms are also indispensable.

6. Typical administrative responsibilities include greeting clients, managing communications, scheduling appointments, triaging clients, and billing. Clinical responsibilities may include client interviews, assisting with medical examinations, taking vital signs, and educating clients.

7. Membership in a professional organization offers a wealth of benefits, including opportunities for ongoing education, links to employment opportunities, and networking with other members of the profession.

8. All work experience is valuable in developing transferable skills. Volunteering is an excellent way to develop skills and build your résumé while contributing to the community and showing your personal commitment.

9. Some colleges have a simulated medical office component integrated into the medical office administration program and some colleges have a cooperative or workplace experience that allows students to apply their learning in a controlled environment. The college, employer, and student all have rights and obligations.

Key Terms

ALLIED HEALTH CARE 6	CORE COMPETENCY 12	PRECEPTOR 21
ALTERNATIVE HEALTH CARE (COMPLEMENTARY HEALTH CARE) 6	EXTERNSHIP 19	REGULATED PROFESSION 17
ATTRIBUTE 8	HEALTH OFFICE PROFESSIONAL 12	SCOPE OF PRACTICE 22
CLIENT 2	LICENSURE 17	TRANSCRIPTION 4
CLIENT 2	MEDICAL ASSISTANT 5	TRIAGE 10
CLINIC 7	MEDICAL OFFICE ASSISTANT 5	WARD CLERK 4

Review Questions

1. How have the duties and responsibilities of the health office professional changed over the past 10 or 20 years, both in the hospital and in the health office setting?

2. Differentiate between attributes and skills. Identify and discuss three attributes and three skills that are important in health office administration.

3. Define professionalism, and discuss what it means for the health-care professional.

4. What is meant by the term *triage*? How does effective triage relate to good judgment?

5. What are the main benefits of remaining calm in an emergency?

6. What are the main advantages of belonging to a professional organization?

7. What is the purpose of a medical office simulation component an externship or cooperative placement experience?

8. Compare and contrast the responsibilities and expectations of the student and the employer during a co-op or workplace experience.

9. What does working within your scope of practice mean?

10. List the benefits of ongoing education for the health office professional.

Application Exercises

1. Review the list of possible employment opportunities for the health office professional. Add any others that you can think of or that are available in your community. Select two or three that interest you. Either individually or in a small group, list the duties and responsibilities you think would apply to each. Over the next week, interview individuals who work in these or similar settings, or research the jobs on the Internet or at the library. Add any new information to your original list. Share your findings with the class.

2. Identify volunteer opportunities available in your community in the following settings (or in settings in which you would like to work). For each, describe the types of volunteer placement you would seek.

   a. A pediatrician's office
   b. A Medical Records Department
   c. An active client-care unit in a hospital

3. Read the following scenario:

   Shauna was doing her cooperative experience in an obstetrical client-care unit that was combined with a neonatal special care unit. The nurse in the special care nursery asked Shauna to watch the unit for her for two minutes while she went to the washroom. She was the only nurse in the unit, and there was no one on the floor that could help. The other two nurses in the client-care unit were attending to a client who had fallen down. There was only one baby in the unit, who was off the respirator, stable, and sleeping. Shauna had an uncomfortable feeling about the situation but hesitantly agreed. The nurse was out of the unit for about a minute when the baby's heart monitor alarm went off. The baby's heart rate had dropped dangerously, and his breathing was laboured. Shauna ran over to the baby. He was blue. Shauna screamed for the nurse, who, fortunately, re-entered the nursery at that moment.

   Discuss this situation. Was Shauna working within her scope of practice? Why, or why not? List alternative courses of action that Shauna could have taken. What would you have done?

4. Construct a resumé suitable for applying for a part-time job, an externship, or a volunteer position. Ask the resource people available at your college to critique your resumé and suggest improvements. Keep this resumé in a file folder. Add all of your course outlines (learning outcomes) to this folder along with assignments that you are proud of.

5. The following exercise is designed to help you identify the attributes you can bring to a job. This will help you set goals, present your strengths in a job interview, and develop a plan to build new strengths.

   a. In small groups, or as a class, discuss each professional quality identified in this chapter as important for health office professionals. Add others that you feel are relevant. Analyze each quality, and list specific examples/situations where you feel that quality would be an asset.

   b. From the above list, select some personal qualities that you think you possess. Under each quality, write a brief summary of ways in which you demonstrate that quality, including examples. Consider achievements you are proud of, whether in school, volunteer work, family life, or hobbies. What personal qualities, strengths, and motivators were instrumental in helping you achieve? Now, ask a classmate or friend to select from the list qualities that she thinks you possess. How do the two descriptions differ? Can you explain these differences? Do you feel you are looking at yourself realistically? Do you come across differently to others from the way you see yourself?

   c. Compare your list and your friend's list with the list of qualities from part a. Are there qualities you need to improve? Prepare a list of strategies.

   d. Identify three people you admire, whether they are people you know personally or public figures. Why do you admire these people? List the qualities you admire in them. Are they qualities you feel you have or ones you would like to develop?

Others will think of a list of possibly serious conditions and may research possible causes. They may be thinking, "This could be serious. I am probably coming down with..." or, "I'll give it a bit more time." At this point, an element of denial remains.

2. Acknowledgment Phase: Sustained Clinical Signs

If the signs persist, perhaps becoming more definite and troublesome, the person will become more concerned. At this stage, the altered health patterns cannot be ignored, and most people feel the need to confide in someone, to seek guidance, and perhaps to validate their own suspicions. They may want someone to reassure them that nothing is wrong, at the same time feeling the need for further action. They often confide in someone close to them and/or someone they trust. It may be an acquaintance who is a health professional. If the perceived condition is potentially serious, an element of denial is more likely to persist. The person may attempt to rationalize symptoms: "I have stomach cramps because of all the aspirin I took last week." "I was at the cottage and probably picked up something from the water there." "This chest pain is probably just indigestion. I should avoid those hamburgers." The client may attempt self-treatment, perhaps with alternative remedies or over-the-counter (OTC) medications. The short-term response is to wait and see. If clinical signs continue, the person will proceed to the next phase.

3. Action Phase: Sustained Clinical Signs

Initial

The next step is to contact a primary health-care provider, usually the family doctor. At this point, the person has admitted that something is, or may be, wrong but has little idea of what is wrong or how serious it is. At this stage, people may be unwilling to face the possibility of a major change in their health, not so much because of fear of illness itself as because they cannot cope with having to change their daily routines and roles.

Subsequent

Following contact with the health-care provider, the person becomes actively involved in seeking concrete information and a diagnosis. Through the process of describing clinical signs and history to the provider, the person acknowledges the altered health pattern and is prepared to investigate probable causes. She becomes actively involved, cognitively and otherwise, in seeking a diagnosis.

4. Transitional Phase: Diagnosis and Treatment

Initial

Response to a diagnosis varies. If it is a simple problem, easily and quickly treated, the person will typically accept the diagnosis and begin the recommended treatment. If the diagnosis is more serious, resulting in protracted treatment, with an undesirable or unpredictable prognosis, acceptance may be delayed. The person may seek a second opinion and/or experience denial, anger, and bargaining before coming to accept it. Some people never accept a really frightening diagnosis. This refusal often has a devastating effect on the family.

Subsequent

Once having accepted the diagnosis, the client considers treatment options offered, makes a choice, and starts treatment. Most providers will invite the individual to participate in any necessary decision making. Often, the provider will explain treatment options and advantages and disadvantages, will make recommendations, but will let the client make the final decision. More decisions may be needed as treatment continues: for example, if the condition does not respond to the initial treatment, the client and doctor may need to reassess and decide whether to try a different treatment. Decisions are rarely purely medical. Other factors come into play, such as pain or inconvenience, cost, time (how long a client has to wait for treatment and how long treatment may take the client from normal activities), emotional factors (such as fear or distaste), and the effects of treatment on family members. Thus, family members may also be involved in making decisions.

5. Resolution Phase: Recovery/Rehabilitation

Once treatment is initiated, the individual's focus shifts to recovery. If the problem is transient, treatment is usually short term, and the client quickly returns to his former position on the health–illness continuum. If the problem is more protracted, the client will continue to focus on recovery. Recovery does not always mean a return to the former health state. For example, a client facing a chronic illness may reach a resolution that involves some limitations and a change in lifestyle. Dealing with this new state takes some adjustment. Over time, most people do come to accept their altered health state. Others fluctuate between acceptance and denial and perhaps may never come to terms with what has happened to them. In the most serious cases, despite treatment, the final resolution may be death. This, too, often involves a series of stages, from learning the prognosis, through denial and anger or bargaining, to acceptance. When the client faces long-term disability or death, family members, too, need to go through a process of assimilating the information and learning to accept it and rebuild their lives.

Implications for the Health Office Professional

By the time a client calls the doctor's office for an appointment, he or she has acknowledged that a health issue exists, and most will be feeling some level of stress about their health state. A cheerful, positive, and caring manner will go a long way to comfort the client. If you sense that the client's condition warrants prompt attention or that the client is very anxious, try to schedule an early appointment (see Chapter 9). In prioritizing appointments, a client's emotional state can be as important as the physical complaint.

Clients who are diagnosed with a serious illness understandably experience protracted stress and display different coping mechanisms. Some clients are initially in complete denial. "It's a mistake. Those test results can't be accurate. We should repeat them." Or, "This can't really be happening. I can't believe it's happened to me. I've done nothing to deserve this." The information they have been given may not register. Other clients may know, in their minds, what the doctor has told them but may not believe it on an emotional level. Some clients may want a second opinion. It is usually not that they do not trust the doctor; they just want another chance at finding out there has been a mistake. Others may believe the diagnosis but want a second opinion just to be sure. If they ask you to make an appointment with another physician gently refer them back to the doctor. Explain that this is something they must discuss with the doctor and that they must have a physician's referral to see another physician. While a second opinion is sometimes a good idea—and doctors themselves will sometimes ask for one—provincial health plans may not cover seeing a physician for a second opinion if the doctor does not feel it is necessary.

Be sensitive to the client's mood and emotional state. The range of responses is wide. A client may not respond at all. He may pick up his belongings, smile, and leave the office. Another client, usually pleasant and talkative, may become just the opposite. A client may appear preoccupied, inattentive, or angry and resentful. Do not take such responses personally. Do your best to remain pleasant, empathetic, and helpful.

The Sick Role and Illness Behaviour

People assume social **roles** in life: positions that carry expectations of responsibilities and of appropriate behaviour. Every person has duties and responsibilities or certain role functions. We have jobs and tasks we must perform, obligations to fulfill, and people who rely on us. Occupational roles determine how a manager and an employee should act; family roles determine how a mother, father, child, or sibling should act. Each of us plays more than one role in life. For example, Bob has roles as a father, a husband, and a teacher. As a father, he has responsibilities to his children. As a husband, he has responsibilities to his wife. As a teacher, he has responsibilities to his colleagues, his employer, and his students. Bob has also taken on roles as a member of the board of his local library and as a scout leader, each of which involves certain obligations.

ROLE   a position in life that carries expectations of responsibilities and of appropriate behaviour.

When people become sick, they are, to varying degrees, excused from their normal roles. When ill, it is acceptable for Bob not to go to work, not to play ball with his children, not to lead his scout troop on a hike. In fact, being sick itself may be considered a role.[6] A person taking on this role, while exempt from normal responsibilities, is expected to behave in certain ways: to rest, to seek professional assistance, and to follow doctor's advice. So far, this behaviour is adaptive. However, the **sick role** can become ineffective. Some people develop a passive, submissive pattern of behaviour that may be quite unlike their normal attitude. This response is more common with serious illness but can also occur in response to minor health problems. Some people seem to have continuous ailments and expect others to wait on and care for them. Others take on a passive role in the face of serious health problems perhaps because of stress, fear, or uncertainty. They may prefer a physician or other health professional to make decisions for them because they trust that person's knowledge and experience or because the loss of their own familiar roles has undermined their sense of autonomy.

SICK ROLE   a particular social role that an ill person adopts, which involves giving up normal responsibilities and accepting care. May sometimes involve uncharacteristically passive behaviour.

This abdication of responsibility is most common when a client is hospitalized, perhaps because of the unfamiliar and highly controlled environment. When you are dependent on others for your food, your mobility, and even your toileting, it can be hard to feel in control of your own life. A client who, to all appearances, becomes immobilized by illness is difficult to deal with for both health professionals and family. The expectations placed on family members are overwhelming. The client may become so passive that she will not participate in her treatment, which impedes recovery. Health professionals must be careful not to cultivate client dependence and should encourage the client to be actively involved in disease prevention, health maintenance, and the treatment of their own illnesses.

Always be sensitive to clients' responses to illness. Recognize that they may need support and encouragement. If a client is cranky or whiny, be patient. If a client seems angry and wants to blame others, be tolerant (within reason). Try to relate the behaviour to the nature, stage, and severity of the client's illness.

---

6.   The concept of the sick role was first developed by sociologist Talcott Parsons as part of an attempt to define health and illness within a general theory of social action. Parsons, T. 1951. *The Social System.* Glencoe, IL: Free Press. Cited in Soma Hewa, "Physicians, the Medical Profession, and Medical Practice," in B. Singh Bolaria and Harley D. Dickinson, eds., *Health, Illness, and Health Care in Canada.* 3rd ed. Scarborough: Nelson Thomson Learning.

Effects on Others

Response to illness is not confined to the person who is ill. Everyone who is closely associated with the sick person will be affected to some extent, both because of concern and because of the effects on their own lives. Spouses and children are especially affected. How much the family is affected will depend on which family member is ill, how serious and how long the illness is, and what cultural and social customs that family has.

As discussed above, a sick person's role changes. This starts a chain reaction, affecting everyone who depends in any way on him. The severity of the effects depends on the nature and seriousness of the illness, as well as on the relationship to the sick person. For example, if Bob became ill, the school would have to bring in a supply teacher. His students might become restless or ill at ease with a new teacher, and the principal might be concerned that the supply teacher was not covering the curriculum. Bob's wife, Nancy, would have to assume the role of both mother and father until Bob recovered. She might also have to take on a new role of caregiver to Bob, perhaps looking after him at home or visiting him in hospital. If his illness was extended, she could find herself increasingly stressed because of the demands on her time and emotional energy and also, perhaps, because of loss of income.

Now consider Katya, a 35-year-old mother of three children. Her husband, Greg, is an electrician. Katya works part time for a busy obstetrician. She is a Girl Guide leader. She accompanies the church choir and is on the board of the library. Each of Katya's roles carries with it responsibilities, and there are people in each of those areas who depend on Katya to carry out those responsibilities.

Let us suppose that Katya comes down with bronchitis. The doctor prescribes an antibiotic and advises Katya to take a few days off. She calls her office to say she will not be in. She has to miss a library board meeting, which she was to chair. She has to cancel choir practice because they have no other pianist. She has to miss a Girl Guide field trip, which means the troop will be short one chaperone and must cancel the event. She is unable take the kids to school or to pick them up. Greg has to get the kids their breakfast and drive them to school, making him an hour late for work. Greg must also pick up the kids from school and put them to bed. He therefore must cancel an important meeting and miss his weekly golf game the next evening. The kids are whiny and clingy because they miss their mother's attention. Dad does not know that Jamie likes porridge for breakfast, and he does not read the right kind of bedtime stories. Katya is not only in discomfort, she feels helpless and frustrated because she is bereft of her normal roles and guilty that she is letting everyone down. Greg is frustrated and feeling inadequate because the kids are not satisfied with the way he does things. He feels somewhat resentful that he has to miss his meeting and golf game. His supervisor is not happy that he came in late, which delayed an important job. The choir members feel under-rehearsed for their next performance. The library board is concerned because it postpones voting on an important matter until the next month…and on it goes.

These examples show how illness affects not just the ill person, but everyone in that person's circle, especially the family. Effects on the family may include

- changes in a person's duties and responsibilities,
- increased stress due to anxiety related to the illness,
- conflict over unaccustomed responsibilities,
- financial problems,
- change in social patterns,
- loneliness (if the family member is hospitalized), and
- pending loss (if the illness is very serious).

from visiting physicians. Clients with health problems that cannot be managed locally are transported, perhaps by air ambulance, to distant medical centres offering a wider range of medical services. People from remote communities may find this sudden appearance in a busy hospital intimidating. They also face the stress of being away from their own familiar environment as well as from the support of family and friends.

The Hospital Environment

To most of us, hospitals, nursing homes, and other client-care facilities are a familiar part of the health-care landscape. Admission to an acute care hospital is fairly common, depending on the nature of the illness. Moving to a nursing home is becoming the norm for elderly people who can no longer care for themselves and whose families cannot provide for them.

To some cultures, however, health-care agencies, whether acute care or long term, are frightening and unwelcome. Koreans, for example, may view admission to hospital as an imminent sign of death and a disharmony with the life forces of yin and yang. Many ethnic minorities will avoid hospitals at all costs, preferring to manage their illnesses at home.

Continued nursing care in a health-care facility poses even greater problems. The thought of entering a nursing home, particularly for cultures where the norm is to care for the elderly at home, is often repugnant. Asian cultures, such as the Vietnamese, typically have a tradition of caring for elderly family members at home, hospitalization being a last resort. An elderly person may avoid or refuse hospitalization, fearing separation from family. Yet, in Canada, attempts to keep an elderly or ill family member at home may become problematic. Family members, despite their cultural norms, may be struggling with full-time jobs and raising a family as well as the stress of bridging two cultures. If they cannot manage with home care and other community support initiatives, the feeling of failure is two-fold: family members may feel they have not fulfilled their responsibilities, and the client admitted to care may feel abandoned.

The pace of the hospital routine in itself may upset the client. Many cultures, for example, Latin Americans, take a more relaxed approach to life in general. They like to take their time, to have things explained, and to consider alternatives. The hectic pace of the hospital may so intimidate and confuse them that they may find it difficult to participate in their own health care. Likewise, in the health office, they may not accept the urgency of a test and may try to fit it into their schedule, rather than rearranging their schedule.

Professionals' Attitudes and Lack of Knowledge

For the health-care system to be fully effective, professionals must understand and adapt to the varied mix of cultural, racial, socioeconomic, and generational differences within their practices. This is a complex undertaking, however, that cannot be achieved overnight. Lack of understanding may lead professionals to be condescending to clients or to otherwise treat them in a way they find disrespectful. Someone with a history of being discriminated against will be quick to perceive any slight and will be hurt. Even a simple error or misunderstanding can lose the client's trust. At worst, the relationship is so impaired that even clients' simple needs are not met.

Differences in Beliefs and Practices

Clients come to a health office bringing varied expectations, shaped by a blend of their culture and their experiences. A person who grew up with a very different health-care system may be surprised at how things are done and may not understand much of what is done and why. People's culturally based beliefs also influence both their decision to seek treatment and their expectations of treatment. This section outlines a few culturally based attitudes that may affect health care. Keep in mind that these are very general. You should never assume that all members of cultural minorities will share the same beliefs, practices, and attitudes. This approach is stereotyping and likely to lead to misunderstandings. Not only do cultures vary, but individuals vary too. Your own attitudes toward health might be quite different from your sister's or your best friend's, and they may change over the course of your lifetime as a result of your own life experiences. Be alert to differences in how individuals approach health care; be aware of their expectations, their compliance with medical treatment, and their understanding of issues affecting their health and treatment.

Recent newcomers (especially younger people) may adopt typical Western health beliefs, values, and expectations very quickly. Others may incorporate a blend of Western beliefs and behaviours with those of their native country, while still others do not embrace Western culture at all. First- and second-generation Canadians are often at odds with their parents and grandparents regarding health beliefs and behaviours. This may promote disharmony within the family. You may at times feel that you are caught in the middle, attempting to honour the rights of the client as well as those of the parents.

Confidentiality

The issue of confidentiality can be complicated by cultural expectations. It is not unusual for a parent to come into the office and demand confidential information about her teenage child or demand that a plan of care for a son or daughter be withdrawn or changed. In some cultures, it is expected that a parent will have access to this type of information, whereas in Canada the matter is usually between the teenage client and the provider. A grown child may come in demanding information about an elderly parent. In some cultures, it is expected that the eldest son, for example, will assume responsibility for care of the parent and therefore have the right to all medical information. In Canada, the exchange of this type of information is not permitted without the client's express permission. In such circumstances, it is best to remain neutral and to discuss the issue with the doctor.

The Philosophy of Prevention

As we discussed in Chapter 2, a preventive model of health care currently predominates in Western culture. Individuals are encouraged to take responsibility for their own wellness. Virtually every community, in partnership with various levels of government, has agencies that promote health education and adaptive lifestyles. Doctors and other health-care professionals have also assumed responsibility for health teaching related to health promotion. Members of some minorities may resist or may not understand this approach. Some cultures, such as those of some First Nations, see health and illness as matters of the here and now. Visiting the doctor's office for an annual physical examination (as is recommended in many provinces) is not a standard practice. This is not deliberate noncompliance or disregard for one's health, just a different perspective. Carefully explain to the client the reasons for the examination. If this does not change the client's attitude and behaviour, you may simply have to respect her perspective. Remember that you can accept and respect a person's point of view without agreeing with it.

The Concept of Illness and Treatment

Many cultures do not accept the concept of chronic illness. When people in these cultures feel better, they consider that the illness has been cured; if they feel poorly again, they consider that a new illness. To someone with this attitude, it is difficult to explain the cycle of **remission** and **exacerbation** that characterizes illnesses such as multiple sclerosis (MS). With MS, there are usually periods when the client feels better (remission) and may be completely symptom free. This is usually the result of a well-established treatment regime. Even with treatment, clinical signs or symptoms will generally reappear (exacerbation). Treatment is adjusted, and perhaps the client will enjoy another remission. Clients who do not see this cycle as part of a chronic illness often stop taking their medication as soon as they feel well, which interferes with effective management of the disease. Consider a client, Ana, with a urinary tract infection for which the physician has prescribed an antibiotic four times a day for 10 days. The doctor assumes she will take the medication as prescribed. As expected, the clinical signs disappear in a day or two. Four days later, Ana calls with complaints that should have been managed by the medication. As soon as Ana felt better, she assumed that she was cured and stopped taking the medication. The way to prevent this problem is to give clients a careful, detailed explanation of the importance of taking the medication until it is finished, even when they no longer experience the signs, and to invite questions to make sure the clients understand.

> **REMISSION**   the phase of a chronic disease characterized by a relief or absence of clinical signs or symptoms.
>
> **EXACERBATION**   the phase of a chronic disease characterized by a return of clinical signs or symptoms.

Different Explanatory Systems

Some cultures have systems of traditional or folk medicine that explain health and illness according to principles different from those of modern Western medicine. Some link health and illness with the supernatural or spiritual world. Some African Canadians, for example, believe in a direct connection between the body and the forces of nature. They may consider propitious dates, stars, and numbers in booking appointments or making decisions about their health care. Traditional Chinese medicine explains health and illness largely in terms of opposing principles. For example, some foods and some conditions are considered "hot" and others "cold." These terms do not refer to temperature but to inherent qualities of substances. People with a "hot" condition are advised to eat "cold" foods and vice versa. You cannot really ask clients whether they believe in magic or in folk medicine, but you can find out about their beliefs by asking what they think is the cause of their symptoms. Such beliefs may influence anything from the food they eat to their level of activity and when they bathe. Respect where they are coming from. Remember that Western medicine does not know everything. Whether or not health beliefs have any basis in fact, people are more likely to do well if they are confident and comfortable with their treatment. Comply with their requests whenever possible. In some cases, you may need to accept that the client will not choose the treatment the health-care provider deems best. There is no universal formula that will allow you to resolve the difference, but remember that the foundation of good health care is respect for the individual. Ultimately, it is the client's health and the client's decision.

Attitudes toward Mental Illness

Mental illness still carries a certain stigma in Western society. For example, although depression is a widespread diagnosis, and anti-depressants are commonly used, many people are reluctant to admit the diagnosis or the use of medication even to friends and family. Individuals with such diseases as bipolar disorder (manic-depression) or schizophrenia are to some extent ostracized. This stigma is even stronger among people, such as some Vietnamese Canadians, whose culture perceives mental illness to be governed by spiritual entities. Hispanics will also often avoid seeking treatment for psychiatric illnesses, feeling that such issues are personal and should be discussed only with family members. Be tolerant, understanding, accepting, and discreet with these clients and their family members when discussing related tests, treatment times, and when booking referral appointments.

Culture and the Health–Illness Continuum

Recall the various definitions of health discussed in Chapter 2. Keep in mind that definitions vary from person to person and culture to culture. In cultures that emphasize a role in the social network, the definition of health may include family relationships and economic roles. Some Asian Canadians, for example, would not consider themselves healthy if they were unable to provide for their families.

To see the effects of differing concepts of health, consider two middle-aged men who become paraplegic after an accident. Sandy, who is a third-generation Canadian of Scottish ancestry, is initially devastated, but after a period of adjustment he feels lucky to be alive. He cannot return to his former work in construction, but after rehabilitation he retrains and is able to do part-time data entry. Even with a disability pension, his income is much lower than before, and his wife must work full time to support the family. However, working from home gives him the satisfaction of spending more time with his children. Before long, he comes to terms with his disability and is able to get on with his life. He considers himself a healthy, productive individual and places himself toward the good health end of the health–illness continuum (see Chapter 2). Lee Wong, who has been in Canada for three years, suffers a similar disability. His limited English skills, however, give him fewer options to retrain. Although he too eventually manages to make a little money, he is devastated at being unable to support his family. He will never consider himself healthy again. Placement on the continuum, for him, remains stationary or moves toward the poor health end of the scale. His doctor and others involved in his care become frustrated at his apparent apathy. They consider that he is feeling sorry for himself and begin to lose patience and interest in him. Lee senses their disrespect, and it enforces his own feelings of inadequacy. Understanding the root of his responses would motivate health professionals to seek another and more effective rehabilitation approach; although difficulties might persist, at least their empathy would help restore some of his self-esteem.

End-of-Life Issues

Advanced technology makes it possible to prolong life for terminally ill clients. Some individuals want every measure possible used to sustain life; others advocate little or no intervention. These decisions reflect cultural, religious, and experientially acquired beliefs and practices. Muslims, for example, generally find it unacceptable to prolong life with machinery unless the individual will be able to lead a satisfactory life.

The death of a family member affects families of different cultures in various ways. The Vietnamese may mourn a loved one for up to three years. They do not usually allow autopsies, believing that the body should remain intact. They may also be reluctant to register as organ donors.

Child Care

In contemporary Western society, mothers often work full time outside the home, relegating child care to a hired nanny or a daycare centre. While many women make this

Payment of Premiums

In Canada, there are two models for the payment of provincial and territorial premiums: (1) residents pay insurance premiums; and (2) the government covers health-care costs through blended taxation.

Only Alberta, British Columbia, and most recently Ontario residents pay insurance premiums. In all other provinces and territories, health care is paid for by tax money from the federal, provincial, and municipal governments, including sales taxes, employer levies, and property taxes. Coverage is universal for legal residents, regardless of employment status.

Alberta

Residents of Alberta must pay Alberta Health Premiums. Rates vary for individual or family coverage. Subsidies are available, under two programs, for those who are unable to pay premiums. The Premium Subsidy Program is based on the previous year's income tax return, while the Waiver of Premiums Program is based on the current financial situation. Residents may be billed monthly or quarterly by mail or may pay by pre-authorized monthly withdrawal. There are penalties for late payments. Beneficiaries receive regular monthly statements. Some employers pay premiums. Seniors, their spouses and dependents, and people aged 55 to 64 receiving the Alberta Widows' Pension receive additional benefits at no cost through the Alberta Blue Cross.

British Columbia

Residents pay premiums, which vary with family size, to the Medical Services Plan (MSP). Premiums must be paid one month in advance, and rates are subject to change. **Beneficiaries** may pay directly to the MSP or through payroll or pension deduction. Canadian citizens and permanent residents living in Canada for the past year may apply for premium assistance based on income. Depending on adjusted net income, they will pay from 20 to 100 percent of the full rate. However, care is not denied to people who fail to pay premiums. There are no premiums for insured hospital services. There is a per diem charge for extended-care hospital services for residents over age 19.

Note that in both B.C. and Alberta, a resident would not be denied necessary medical care because of nonpayment of premiums.

BENEFICIARY a person eligible to receive insurance benefits under specified conditions.

Health-Care Delivery

Several models of health-care delivery and remuneration are used in Canada. Most physicians work in private (solo) or group practices independent of the government. Some work in educational facilities/hospitals, clinics, community health centres, or family health networks. Although several methods of payment are used, the majority of physicians in Canada are paid on a fee-for-service basis. This is changing, however, with the introduction of various primary care reform initiatives across the country.

Health-care structures and settings are quite similar across Canada, both in and out of hospital. Across Canada, these structures are under review. What services should be covered? Who should deliver them? These questions are continually re-examined in search of a balance between cost and quality.

Primary Health Care

Primary health care is the provision of integrated health-care services by providers who address the majority of a client's health concerns. Primary health care also refers

PRIMARY HEALTH CARE (1) integrated health care by a provider who addresses the majority of a client's health concerns; (2) treatment administered during the first medical contact for a health concern.

to treatment administered during the first medical contact for a particular health concern. Usually, family physicians (also called family practitioners) deliver primary care, sometimes along with a team of health professionals, such as nurse practitioners and physiotherapists. In Canada, specialists are not considered primary care providers because a client must have a referral from a family doctor.

Although physicians within a *family practice* provide *primary care*, the terms are not interchangeable. Family physicians provide a range of services well beyond the scope of what is defined as primary care services. Emergency Departments or urgent-care clinics provide primary care in emergencies but do not provide the full range of services offered in a family practice.

The **family physician** (also called a family doctor or general practitioner) is an MD (medical doctor) whose postgraduate specialty is in family medicine. Family physicians are generalists—they look after the general medical needs of clients from babies to seniors. Primary care includes health promotion, disease prevention, health maintenance, counselling, patient education, and diagnosis and treatment of acute and chronic illnesses in a variety of health-care settings (e.g., office, hospital, critical care, long-term care, home care, daycare). Primary care is performed and managed by a family physician, often collaborating with other health professionals and using consultation or referral as appropriate.

Primary care, in the sense of care at point of contact, is also provided by specialists in emergency medicine, or **emergentologists**.

A **locum tenens**, often simply called a "locum," is a doctor temporarily taking over another doctor's practice, such as during vacations. If the practice is specialized, the locum must have the same specialty. Primary care physicians often use a locum when they travel.

Specialists and Primary Care

Specialists (also called consultants) are not considered primary care physicians, although some specialists do render some primary care services. (For example, obstetricians provide the same type of prenatal primary care assessments that family physicians do; clients are referred to them either because they are high risk or because their family physician does not deliver babies.) Clients cannot go directly to a specialist but must be referred by a primary care physician. Most family practitioners quickly realize what conditions they are equipped to handle and when they should refer to a specialist for diagnosis or treatment. For example, Amina went to see her family doctor because of abdominal pain. The doctor conducted a series of tests but could not find the cause. She referred Amina to an internist (specialist in internal medicine) for further investigation. The internist discovered that Amina had gestational diabetes (diabetes during pregnancy) and referred her to an obstetrician for continued assessment. The obstetrician and internist would provide collaborative care for Amina.

Primary Health-Care Settings in Canada

Solo Practice

Solo practice refers to a physician practising independently, with staff members, who may include a health office professional, a nurse, or both. The physician in solo practice may share a call schedule with other doctors to provide extended coverage for clients.

Group Practice

A group practice involves several physicians, who may or may not share office space, expenses, and support staff. Depending on the mix of providers, they may also share a

FAMILY PHYSICIAN   an MD with a specialty in family medicine who looks after the general medical needs of a varied practice population.

EMERGENTOLOGIST   a physician specializing in emergency medicine.

LOCUM TENENS (LOCUM)   a doctor temporarily taking over another doctor's practice.

call schedule. A group practice is usually, but not always, made up of providers within the same specialty. There is frequently a legal arrangement, such as related to billing, but the group may not be incorporated. The physicians may have a group number for provincial billing purposes. Often, the services of the group's physicians are provided through the group, are billed in the name of the group, and the resulting revenues are treated as receipts of the group.

Partnership

Strictly speaking, a partnership is a business formed by two or more individuals who are jointly and separately financially liable for the operation of the business. Some physicians form such legal partnerships. While they submit fee-for-service claims individually and do not have a group billing number, their income, net of expenses, is considered by Revenue Canada to be personal taxable income of individual partners. Other physicians simply share certain expenses of the practice through an informal or formal agreement. Each physician has clearly defined responsibilities, rights, and obligations. Note that physicians will often speak loosely of colleagues with whom they share a call schedule as "partners," although they are not actually members of a partnership.

Professional Corporation

A professional corporation is a legally incorporated business that allows professionals to reap many of the benefits of a for-profit corporation. A medical professional corporation must be organized for the sole purpose of rendering medical services, and the shareholders must be licensed physicians. The corporation may simply handle expenses, with each physician otherwise practising independently. Alternatively, the physicians may be employees of the corporation, along with others such as administrative staff. Services within a corporation vary. They may include physiotherapy, laboratory and diagnostic facilities, and alternative modalities such as acupuncture and chiropractic. The main advantages are financial. Health maintenance organizations (discussed below) are one type of corporation.

Clinics

A clinic is a health-care setting that offers services to outpatients. A clinic can be managed by one physician or by a group of physicians and may offer services ranging from the simple diagnosis and treatment of complaints to therapeutic or preventive treatments. Some clinics offer a range of services under one roof, such as laboratory, physiotherapy, and consultations with specialists. There are also specialty clinics such as prenatal, oncology, or orthopedic. Clinics may be privately owned, government sponsored, or organized by a group of doctors who share space and staff but bill separately. Clinics vary in name and in services offered. The following descriptions are general.

- ◆ *Walk-in clinics* (also called *after-hours clinics* or *ambulatory care clinics*) offer medical services to clients, usually without an appointment. Sometimes, a group of family physicians will offer after-hours care for **orphan patients** (clients who do not have a regular doctor) or for patients who, for whatever reason, could not see their own physician during office hours. A walk-in clinic may or may not treat urgent complaints such as fractures and lacerations.

- ◆ *After-hours clinics*, most typically, are organized by physicians within a community to ease the stress on local Emergency Departments and operated on a fee-for-service basis, with the physicians sharing office and administrative costs. As with walk-in clinics, they are likely to accept any client. (Unlike after-hours clinics operated by formal groups, such as the Family Health Networks (FHNs) and the Family Health Groups (FHGs) in Ontario, where

ORPHAN PATIENT a client who does not have a family physician and must get medical services from clinics and emergency departments.

services are restricted to clients who are rostered with the practice and/or who are clients of the physicians participating in the group.)

- ◆ *Urgent-care clinics* also offer services without an appointment. The main difference is the focus on immediate care of urgent, but not life-threatening complaints, such as lacerations or fractures. An urgent-care clinic may also offer diagnostic and perhaps pharmacy services.

- ◆ *Outpatient clinics*, often located at or connected to a hospital, provide medical services to clients who have been discharged from the facility, as well as to others who need their often specialized services. Clinics may or may not require appointments. Examples of types of outpatient clinics include oncology, diabetic, and orthopedic.

Emergency Department

Emergency departments (emergency rooms, ERs) do provide non-urgent primary care, but they are supposed to be reserved for clients in acute distress, such as chest pain, stroke symptoms (numbness/tingling in a limb; severe headache, visual disturbances) or difficulty breathing. Others are encouraged to see their family physician or seek medical care elsewhere. However, many clients go to ERs for health concerns that could easily be managed elsewhere, exacerbating overcrowding. Educating clients in a general practice setting about appropriate use of an ER is important. This overuse of ERs results partly from the large number of orphan patients across the country. If there are no available ambulatory care clinics, an orphan patient has nowhere else to go.

Not every hospital offers emergency services, and ERs in different hospitals may render different levels of care. Some ERs, for example, lack the capacity to deal with major trauma cases. All hospitals, however, will have procedures in place to direct emergencies, including evacuating clients to appropriate trauma centres. A fully active ER is open 24 hours a day, seven days a week, and is equipped to deal with almost all emergencies.

Managed Care

MANAGED CARE   a set of strategies, procedures, and policies designed to control the use of health-care services, sometimes by organizing doctors, hospitals, and other providers into groups in order to improve the quality and cost-effectiveness of health care.

Primary care settings also include those managed by health organizations, often referred to as managed care organizations. **Managed care** is a set of strategies, procedures, and policies designed to control the use of health-care services. Such strategies include a review of medically necessary services, enticement to use certain providers, and case management. The goal is to conserve health-care expenditure, while maintaining quality, by reorganizing health-care delivery within a community. Managed care techniques are most often practised by organizations and professionals that assume responsibility for the population of a geographic area. Managed care is a broad term and refers to many different types of organizations, methods of remuneration, review mechanisms, and partnerships. Managed care is sometimes used as a general term for the activity of organizing doctors, hospitals, and other providers into groups to improve the quality and cost-effectiveness of health care, as in the primary care reform initiatives discussed later. Medical care is carefully planned to make optimum use of resources. Arrangements often involve a defined delivery system of providers with some form of contractual arrangement with the plan. A health maintenance organization is an example of a managed care organization.

Health Maintenance Organizations (HMOs)

HMOs offer prepaid, comprehensive health coverage for both hospital and physician services. An HMO contracts with qualified physicians, hospitals, and other health professionals. Most commonly, HMOs combine a group practice with a payment or

Saskatchewan Health
http://www.health.gov.sk.ca/

Manitoba Health
http://www.gov.mb.ca/health/mhsip/

Ontario Health and Long-Term Care
http://www.health.gov.on.ca/

Quebec Health
http://www.ramq.gouv.qc.ca/crc/

New Brunswick Department of Health
and Wellness
http://www.gnb.ca/0051/index-e.asp

Nova Scotia Department of Health
http://www.gov.ns.ca/health/

Prince Edward Island Health and Social Services
http://www.gov.pe.ca/hss/index.php3

Newfoundland and Labrador
http://www.gov.nf.ca/mcp/

The Romanow Report
http://www.canada.com/national/features/
     healthcare/
http://www.healthcarecommission.ca/

Useful Definitions Used by Health Canada
http://www.canlii.org/ca/sta/c-6/sec2.html

History of Health Care in Canada
http://www.misc-iecm.mcgill.ca/HCC/pages/
     iecm_section5a.html

Website for Rheophoresis
http://www.rheoclinic.com/consumers/
     rheophoresis/

Part III

Health Care Basics

Part III gets down to basic information about quality and standards, diagnostic testing, and pharmacology that applies to any health-related occupational setting. Chapter 5 introduces the principles of quality, standards, and safety in health care. Essential topics, such as occupational health and safety legislation, WHMIS, asepsis, infection control, and Standard Precautions, are discussed in some detail. You will learn effective risk management techniques appropriate to your role in health care. Environmental safety for both health professionals and clients is also discussed. Chapter 6 will introduce you to diagnostic testing, including laboratory tests and diagnostic imaging, and to your role in the process. You will be instrumental in requisitioning these tests, accurately and responsibly reporting test results to the appropriate people, and booking appointments for clients. You will also inform clients about preparing for tests and about what to expect. Chapter 7 will provide you with a knowledge base about pharmacology suitable to your related responsibilities. You will gain an overview of types of drugs, drug effects and side effects, and routes of administration. You will learn how to deal with prescriptions in the health office and how to direct clients to appropriate resources when they have questions related to their medications.

Standards and Safety in Health Care

On completing this chapter, you will be able to:

1. Discuss the concept of quality assurance in health care.
2. Outline the employer's and employee's responsibilities under occupational health and safety legislation.
3. Explain the purpose and requirements of the Workplace Hazardous Materials Information System.
4. Outline the chain of infection.
5. Describe the properties of five infectious organisms.
6. Differentiate between active immunity and passive immunity.
7. Discuss the principles of asepsis and sterilization applied in the health office.
8. Demonstrate appropriate techniques for removing contaminated gloves.
9. Discuss safety in the health office setting, considering issues related to age and environmental and personal factors.
10. Identify potential sources of injury for the health office professional in the workplace setting, and strategies.
11. Explain the steps to prevent fire and to prepare for possible fires.

When you go to a restaurant, you expect your food to be of high quality, prepared according to certain standards. When you purchase a shirt or a car, you likewise expect the product to reflect a certain quality. Even dealing with a bank, you expect that the individuals who manage your money will be appropriately trained and will know what they are doing. Health care is no different. It is a service; its scope and nature vary, and it is provided by individuals whom you expect to be appropriately trained and knowledgeable. You also expect the services you receive to be of a certain quality. As a health office professional, you must be aware of the standards of care and service that your facility and you, yourself, are expected to provide. You must participate in ongoing evaluation and ensure that you maintain a high standard of service.

Quality Assurance in Health Care

Quality assurance is any systematic process of checking to see whether a product or service is meeting requirements. Quality assurance also includes establishing, promoting, and maintaining a safe occupational environment. Industry and other occupational settings embody specific goals and criteria in their quality assurance initiatives. Industrial settings often have a full-time quality control officer.

Quality assurance in the health-care environment is an orchestrated and methodical approach of continuously scrutinizing, evaluating, and improving the quality of health services. Clients should expect nothing short of excellence in assessment, diagnosis,

QUALITY ASSURANCE
any systematic process of checking to see whether a product or service is meeting specified requirements. In health care, it is a systematic assessment to ensure that services are of the highest possible quality using existing resources.

treatment, and ongoing care. They are entitled to prompt treatment, prompt reports on laboratory tests, accurate prescriptions, reasonable waiting times, direction regarding emergencies, and proper follow-up. Quality assurance is particularly critical when budgets are limited and resources scarce.

Quality assurance in health care is the responsibility of both employers and employees. Large facilities usually have a formal quality assurance committee. In small practices, you, as the health office professional, play a large role. To do so effectively, you must understand the principles of quality assurance and safety, including infection control. You must be conscious of both your own and the clients' safety in the office.

It is vital to maintain a safe environment in the health office—one that reduces risk of harm to both clients and staff. In the health office, you will encounter people from all age groups, with varied health problems, altered emotional and physical needs, and a wide range of abilities and disabilities. You have a special responsibility to protect those who cannot effectively protect themselves. You need to protect both yourself and them against injury, fire, and infection.

Hospitals

Hospitals and other health-care facilities participate in a process known as accreditation (discussed in Chapter 14), which demonstrates that they meet provincial/territorial standards. Health-care providers, such as doctors and midwives, must go through a peer-review process of *credentialling* to establish and maintain privileges to admit and care for clients at a health-care facility. Health-care facilities periodically review facility policies, procedures, and quality of care. The following include some of the problems frequently reviewed. Investigations into these areas cover policies, procedures, documentation, and actual client care.

- Clients who are re-admitted to hospital within a certain number of days after discharge
- Deaths occurring within the hospital
- Unscheduled returns to surgery
- Infections contracted within the hospital
- Falls, medication errors, and other irregularities

Investigation will hopefully lead to improved client care.

Health Offices

Many smaller health offices do not have a formal quality assurance plan. If your office does not have such a plan, you may want to propose establishing one. However, quality assurance is addressed informally each time an action is taken to correct a problem or improve services to clients. Remember that a quality assurance plan can only be as good as the people who initiate and practise it. A quality assurance review should follow the following principles:

- In a large enough setting (for example, the health department of a large factory), a committee should be designated to oversee the process. This may require formal training of some or all of the committee members. In a smaller health office with few employees, it is most effective if everyone works as a team.
- Keep it positive. A review is not meant to punish those who make errors, but to find the causes of problems and correct them. Stress the goal of enhancing performance and client service.

◆ Actively involve all staff so that everyone "owns" the process. A collaborative effort generalizes problems, avoids pinpointing blame, and promotes working toward the common goal of improved service and care.

All services in the office should be open to review, with more thorough investigation of trouble spots, such as

◆ errors in writing prescriptions,

◆ mislabelling of test specimens,

◆ multiple needle-sticks by staff,

◆ frequent, long waiting periods for clients in the reception area,

◆ inadequate or delayed follow-up on abnormal test results,

◆ protracted delay in returning phone calls,

◆ not answering the telephone within a reasonable time frame,

◆ inaccurate or incomplete documentation and charting,

◆ errors in letters, reports, and so on,

◆ client concerns about involvement in selecting treatments, and

◆ client concern about the type and length of treatment offered.

Once areas of concern have been identified, measures to address each must be outlined and implemented. Periodic review is needed to assess progress. A suggestion box in the waiting room may help identify client concerns and generate valuable ideas.

The Incident Report

An incident report is formal documentation of any lapse in acceptable procedure, protocol, or policy. Incident reports are more commonly seen in larger agencies such as hospitals and busy clinics. The incident report has long been dreaded as an instrument bringing blame and punishment to those perceived to be responsible. More recently, incident reports have taken on a more positive role, focusing not on assigning blame, but on identifying problems, determining why they occurred, and suggesting corrective steps. Most often, incidents are not the fault of one person but are the result of a combination of events. The incident report also provides detailed and accurate documentation that may be needed for legal purposes.

The format of an incident report will vary with the agency. However, most include

◆ a summary of the event;

◆ a detailed account of events leading up to the incident;

◆ date and time of the event;

◆ who was present initially, and anyone else involved in the incident;

◆ who was notified of the event (e.g., coordinator, clinical leader) and when;

◆ any untoward consequences;

◆ any action, medical or otherwise, taken as a result of the event (e.g., physician ordered an X-ray after a client's fall);

◆ an evaluation of the incident; and

◆ recommendations for preventing a similar occurrence.

Incident reports are a valuable tool for identifying areas of concern. An isolated incident may not raise undue concern. However, if similar incidents happen repeatedly, a thorough investigation of causes is called for. Similarly, when a health professional is injured, a formal report must be completed, detailing the events leading up to, during, and following the occurrence. This report is used to ensure follow-up care and perhaps compensation for the injured worker. The factors causing or contributing to the incident are reviewed and dealt with, either internally or under the direction of an outside body such as the Workers' Compensation Board (WCB), which is discussed later.

International Organization for Standardization (ISO)

The ISO is a worldwide nongovernmental organization of standardization bodies that has produced a set of international standards for a globally accepted quality assurance system. To achieve ISO registration, a company or agency must develop a set of procedures to ensure that its services or products are of high quality and suitable for their intended purpose. ISO registration is reviewed on a regular schedule, at least every five years. The ISO sets standards of safety, identifies reliable suppliers, and helps build client/consumer confidence. Health facilities are major purchasers of goods (such as diagnostic equipment, intravenous supplies, surgical supplies, medications, needles and syringes, dressings, computers, and administrative supplies) and services (such as laundry, dietary, or janitorial). Since reliable excellence is crucial, many health agencies will purchase only from suppliers with the appropriate ISO registration.

The registration process begins when an agency or company fills out an application form. An accredited independent third party conducts an on-site audit of the agency's operations against the applicable ISO standards. The applicant then has time to prepare to meet the standards. After a rigorous assessment and inspection, if all standards are met, the agency or company receives a certificate identifying its product or service as being in compliance with ISO standards. The agency will be listed in a register maintained by an accredited third-party organization.

The application of ISO standards to health-care settings themselves is relatively new. The medical department at the General Motors plant in Oshawa, Ontario, for example, has achieved ISO designation. The ISO designation guarantees that the department's services satisfy its customers—the workforce, the Workplace Safety and Insurance Board (Ontario's equivalent to the Workers' Compensation Board), and other insurance providers. The designation also ensures that the medical manual is current, client records are accurate and up-to-date, customers are given relevant information within a reasonable time frame, and employees have clearly defined roles.

Occupational Health and Safety

All workers face hazards on the job. Health office professionals face the same risks as any office worker—such as safety issues related to equipment and surroundings and the risk of repetitive strain injuries—as well as specific risks related to infection and contamination. These risks are discussed later in the chapter. To protect workers against hazards on the job, all provinces and territories have Occupational Health and Safety (OHS) legislation that outlines the general rights and responsibilities of employers, supervisors, managers, and workers. The law makes both the employer and the employee jointly responsible for health and safety. You need to know your rights and responsibilities and how to access more information if you need it.

The details of the OHS legislation vary slightly from one jurisdiction to another, but the basic elements are the same.[1]

---

1. Adapted with permission from information provided by the Canadian Centre for Occupational Health and Safety (CCOHCS). 250 Main Street East, Hamilton, Ontario, L8N 1H6, 1-800-283-8466.

The Government's Responsibilities

The government has a responsibility to

- develop and enforce occupational health and safety legislation;
- designate safety officers who inspect workplaces to ensure compliance;
- disseminate information;
- promote education, training, and research; and
- take action in case of noncompliance.

The Employee's Rights and Responsibilities

The employee has the right to

- refuse unsafe work;
- participate in the workplace health and safety activities through the Joint Health and Safety Committee, or act as the employee health and safety representative; and
- know about actual and potential dangers in the workplace.

The employee has the responsibility to

- comply with the OHS act and regulations,
- use personal protective equipment and clothing as directed by the employer, and
- report workplace hazards and dangers.

The Supervisor's Responsibilities

The supervisor must

- ensure that employees use prescribed protective equipment and devices,
- advise employees of any potential hazards, and
- take reasonable precautions to protect employees.

The Employer's Responsibilities

The employer must

- establish and maintain a joint health and safety committee, or have employees select at least one health and safety representative;
- take every reasonable precaution to ensure that the workplace is safe;
- train all employees about any potential hazards;
- supply personal protective equipment and ensure that employees know how to use it safely and properly;
- immediately report all critical injuries to the Ministry of Labour; and
- train all employees how to safely use, handle, store, and dispose of hazardous substances and how to handle emergencies.

The Joint Health and Safety Committee

Large workplaces are usually required to form a committee to deal with any occupational health issues, which may also be called an Industrial Health and Safety Committee, Occupational Health Committee, Health and Safety Committee, or Workplace Safety and Health Committee. The committee is made up of an equal number of representatives from management and the employees—an employee elected or selected by his union and co-chaired by an employee and a management representative. Committees must meet every three months and are supposed to work cooperatively to identify and solve problems. The committee

- acts as an advisory body,
- identifies hazards and obtains information,
- recommends corrective actions,
- assists in resolving work refusal cases, and
- participates in accident investigations and workplace inspections.

Smaller workplaces may be required to have a health and safety representative.

Work Refusals

An employee can refuse work if she has reason to believe that the situation is unsafe to herself or to co-workers.

- The employee must report to the supervisor/manager that she is refusing work and state why she believes the situation is unsafe.
- The employee, the supervisor/manager, and a Joint Health and Safety Committee (JHSC) member will investigate the situation.
- The employee must return to work when the problem is solved.
- If the problem is not resolved, a government health and safety inspector is called.
- The supervisor/manager may assign the employee other work.
- The inspector will investigate and render a decision.

In addition, Ontario legislation allows a certified member of the Health and Safety Committee to direct the employer to stop work if all of the following conditions exist:

- The health and safety legislation is being violated.
- The violation poses a danger or hazard to employees.
- Any delay in controlling the danger or hazard may seriously endanger an employee.

The Canadian Centre for Occupational Health and Safety provides information useful to both employers and employees in every type of workplace setting, from the health office to the factory environment. Topics include biological hazards; diseases, disorders, and injuries; health and safety programs; prevention and control of hazards; and workplace schedules. Detailed information about these topics and more are available on their Web site (see the list of sites at the end of this chapter.)

The Workplace Hazardous Materials Information System (WHMIS)[2]

Almost all workers who work in an environment other than an office (estimated to be over three million Canadians) are exposed every day to potentially hazardous chemicals on the job. Health office professionals are no exception. For example, a hospital unit may have pure oxygen, which is a highly combustible material. If there is a lab on site, corrosive materials may be a concern. Biohazardous materials are present in some form in most health settings. Even a small health office will have potentially hazardous substances that should be properly labelled and catalogued.

---

2.   This section is adapted from a fact sheet provided by the Ontario WSIB.

Table 5.3 | Minimum Acceptable Vaccination Schedule, as Recommended by Health Canada

Age in Months	Vaccine Administered at Separate Injection Sites, Same Visit
2	Pentacel + Prevnar
4	Pentacel + Prevnar
6	Pentacel + Prevnar
12	Menjugate + Prevnar
13 or 14	MMR and Varivax
18	Pentacel

1. Prevnar contains several strains of the pneumococcus bacterium, which can cause ear infections, pneumonia, and bacteremia and can lead to meningitis. This vaccine may be started as early as two months of age. Number of doses required depends on the timing of the first dose.

2. Menjugate is a vaccine for the meningococcal bacterium. This bacterium caused a small epidemic in London, Ontario in 2001. In most jurisdictions, the provincial plan will cover the cost of the vaccine if there is a concern in the community about contracting this infection.

3. Varivax II, released in 1998, is recommended for children over the age of one year who have *not* had chicken pox.

Recommended Immunizations and Tests for Health Professionals

In any health-care setting, you will naturally be exposed to more sick people than in most workplaces. Therefore, you should be immunized against the infections that present common threats. Many people object to vaccinations because they are too busy, they dislike shots, or they misinterpret minor local reactions as allergic reactions. However, immunizations not only protect you, but protect your clients: if you contract an infection, you are likely to pass it on to clients, some of whom are particularly vulnerable.

Check with your doctor to see that your routine immunizations are up-to-date. Some people believe that childhood vaccinations will protect them for life. While this is true with some vaccines, many require boosters to maintain immunity. Many facilities have a specific list of immunizations required for employees and often for volunteers and students on externships. For some diseases, you may have the option of having antibody titres done, which would test for immunity. Some colleges may also require immunizations for health office administration students and will provide opportunities to receive all necessary shots.

INFLUENZA In most parts of the country, the influenza vaccine is readily available, and it is generally recommended that everyone, including children, be immunized. Health-care professionals are at risk for contracting the flu and are potential host reservoirs for passing the infection to someone else.

HEPATITIS A AND B Hepatitis B immunization requires a series of three injections—the second, one month after the first, and the third, six months thereafter. Hepatitis A requires two injections. Some facilities make this immunization a condition of employment. A contraindication is hypersensitivity to yeast.

MEASLES, MUMPS, RUBELLA Anyone who is at risk for contracting these diseases should be immunized. Although most Canadians are immune (older people because they had the diseases as children and younger people from childhood immunizations), another dose may be recommended. Contraindications include pregnancy, receipt of immunoglobulins, or a sensitivity to eggs or neomycin. There is controversy over individuals who have a sensitivity to eggs. Only life-threatening reactions are considered to be a firm contraindication; people with the potential for such reaction can be tested with a weaker version of the serum.

PNEUMOCOCCAL INFECTIONS Although health-care professionals are not considered to be at higher risk than the general population, some facilities recommend this immunization for their employees' own protection. It is particularly recommended for health professionals with such chronic illnesses as diabetes, heart disease, or disorders of the immune system.

DIPHTHERIA/TETANUS/PERTUSSIS Booster shots are recommended every 10 years after primary immunization has been given. Health-care professionals are not considered to be at higher risk than the general population.

TUBERCULIN TESTING Tuberculosis (TB) is a disease that is constantly being monitored. In Canada, after several decades of decline, the annual incidence rate of TB has remained about the same for the last 10 years, with an estimated 1700 to 2000 new cases reported annually. TB is not declining, primarily because of immigration and international travel to and from areas where it is prevalent, including East, Southeast, and Southern Asia; Sub-Saharan Africa; parts of South and Central America; the Caribbean; Eastern Europe; and the former Soviet Union. Aboriginal people also have a higher incidence of TB, as do individuals with HIV and those living in poor economic circumstances.

Most health-care facilities require that health professionals be tested for TB. The most common screening test is called the Mantoux test. It is recommended for individuals in whom active TB is suspected or who are at risk for exposure, such as health-care workers. A small amount of purified protein derived from the tubercle bacillus is injected under the person's skin. After 48 to 72 hours, the test is interpreted according to the amount of redness and swelling (called induration) at the site. A person with a significant reaction (10 mm or more induration) will have follow-up including a history, chest X-ray, and sputum specimens. Delayed reactions can be noted up to two weeks after the test and should be reported to the doctor. To distinguish between a booster response and conversion by new infections, a second test is often done 12 to 21 days after the first.

Preventing the Spread of Infection

The most effective way to break the cycle of infection is to control the transmission of pathogens from one source to another. Although you are not directly involved in client care, your actions can transmit pathogens or prevent their transmission. An understanding of asepsis is essential.

The first line of defence, in both the hospital and the health office, is personal cleanliness. You can easily carry microorganisms into the work setting or back home on your clothing and on your person. If you carry pathogens home, you can become ill or spread illness to your family. If you carry pathogens to the hospital or office, you may spread infection to vulnerable clients. For this reason, some health-care facilities ask direct care staff members to leave their uniforms and shoes at work. Although this policy does not usually apply to administrative staff, it is a good idea. Wearing a uniform or lab coat only at work limits the chance of transmitting harmful organisms both at work and outside. A uniform or lab coat also looks professional, is easy to launder, and protects your own clothes.

Medical Asepsis

Medical **asepsis** is killing germs *after they leave* the body. The purpose is to reduce or control the number of microorganisms; it does not completely eliminate them. We practise medical asepsis in our daily lives every time we wash our hands, use a tissue when we cough or sneeze, or clean countertops with a disinfectant after preparing food. Medical asepsis should be practised in every health-care setting.

THE HEALTH OFFICE The office and reception areas must be kept scrupulously clean at all times. You should provide the office cleaning service with guidelines for cleaning, including the use of disinfectants, as required. The more specific the guidelines, the better. A checklist for the cleaning staff to tick off will ensure that all required areas are cleaned and will document what has been done.

The reception area should be well ventilated, and seating should place clients at a comfortable distance from each other. If possible, have two or three groupings of chairs. Ask clients with known infectious conditions not to visit the office, or if they must be seen, book them at the end of the day. Do not book clients who are susceptible to infections at the same time as someone who may have one, for example, a person who thinks she might have the flu. Having said that, there are times when this information is simply not available. All you can do is your best to keep infectious clients away from others, especially older clients and children. *Note*: Do not book a pregnant client at the same time as someone who might have rubella. The rubella virus can be **teratogenic** to the fetus in the first trimester of pregnancy.

Properly clean all instruments such as stethoscopes, otoscopes, ophthalmoscopes, and thermometers. Some articles must be sterilized and others disinfected (discussed in more detail later in this chapter). Carefully clean the examination rooms between clients. Wipe down the examination bed and counters between clients if you suspect they have an infectious disease or if there has been contamination with any body fluid. Dispose of garbage frequently and properly.

Provide tissues and an adequate number of wastebaskets, and consider putting up a sign asking clients to use tissues when they cough or sneeze. If there are children's toys in the office, they should be the type that can be wiped down daily with a disinfectant. Books for small children are often available in materials that can be wiped clean.

Specimens, such as urine samples, left in the washroom should be handled with gloves. Wipe the counter and any visible spills after a specimen has been removed. Do not leave specimens (e.g., urine) sitting in the washroom where another client may spill them or come in contact with them.

HEALTH-CARE FACILITIES Follow the principles outlined above, as well as facility guidelines on specific situations. Nosocomial infection is a serious problem in hospitals, leading to considerable morbidity and mortality, particularly among clients who are coping with other illnesses or recovering from surgery.

The janitorial staff cleans most hospital areas thoroughly and regularly. They almost always wear gloves. Garbage cans are emptied frequently, and all areas, including clients' rooms, are dusted and wiped. A thorough *terminal cleaning* is done when a client is discharged.

Staff members who have potentially infectious diseases are encouraged not to come to work, and the general public with infectious conditions are asked not to visit hospitalized clients. Staff members in some facilities are required to receive the flu vaccine annually and keep other required immunizations current. This can be a contentious issue for employees who do not wish to have the flu vaccine, but most hospitals are firm about this policy.

When a facility imposes visiting restrictions, you may be required to inform visitors and to help enforce restrictions. It is not uncommon for long-term care facilities

ASEPSIS   a state in which pathogens are absent or reduced. There are two principal types of asepsis: medical and surgical.

TERATOGENIC   causing abnormalities in the fetus.

to be quarantined if there is an outbreak of the flu or other infectious disease. This may include a total ban on visitors to a single client-care unit or to the entire facility. Such events are stressful for everyone. Clients become anxious about illness and miss the contact with family and friends. They may become demanding and bad tempered. Family members may dismiss the need for **quarantine** and insist on visiting. They may be upset, argumentative, rude, and sometimes even aggressive. Staff are caught in the middle and may also be coping with increased workloads and longer workdays if some of the staff are ill. Infected clients may be isolated (see discussion later) in an attempt to contain the infection.

QUARANTINE isolating or separating a client, client-care unit, or facility.

Hand Washing

Hand washing is probably the single most important component of medical asepsis and the single most effective method of protecting yourself and others from infection. How often you wash your hands will depend on the scope of your nonadministrative duties. Wash your hands after breaks and before and after preparing an examination room, assisting with a procedure, or assisting a client. Wash them before and after using gloves or handling specimens, waste, or potentially soiled instruments or other articles. Figure 5.3 illustrates the proper hand-washing technique.

To wash your hands, properly, you need

◆ soap,
◆ running water,
◆ a clean towel, and
◆ a garbage can.

It really does not matter what type of soap you use. Soaps and detergents are not disinfectants. They emulsify, reducing surface tension to facilitate the removal of soil and organisms. Hands can be cleaned but never sterilized and will always harbour some organisms. Follow these steps:

1. Remove all jewellery, such as rings and watches, as these items can harbour bacteria and other organisms, preventing effective washing. Also, look for breaks in your skin, which provide a portal of entry/exit for organisms. If there are any, it is best to wear gloves.

2. Turn on water, and adjust to a comfortable temperature.

3. Add enough cleansing agent to your hands to create suds.

4. Wet hands, rubbing all areas vigorously. Ensure that you clean nails, fingers, between your fingers, and the front and back of the hands up to the wrist area. Nails need special attention, as do the areas between your fingers. Nail polish, especially if chipped, will also provide a hiding place for organisms. If you frequently touch clients, instruments, or other articles used in client care, it is a good idea not to wear nail polish in the office and to keep your nails reasonably short.

5. Scrub, using good friction, for one to two minutes.

6. Rinse off all soap, preferably by putting your hands under the running water fingers first and moving your hands up under the running water.

7. Dry your hands, again beginning at your fingertips and patting them dry up to the wrist.

8. Using the towel, turn off the taps.

9. Discard the soiled towel.

Remember: It is the friction and the running water that does the job.

♦ If the eyes or other mucous membranes are exposed, flush clean with sterile water, saline, or a sterile irrigant.

♦ Notify your immediate supervisor promptly.

Fill out a WCB accident report form. The occurrence should be reported to the manager of the facility or office, the occupational health coordinator, and the employee health department, if these exist, and your Ministry of Health.

Decisions must then be made—quickly—about **postexposure prophylaxis (PEP)**. If the source person is willing to be tested, obtain consent and initiate appropriate diagnostic tests promptly. If the source person refuses testing, consider her risk factors. If the source person is in a low-risk category, the contaminated person may choose to forgo treatment. This must be a personal decision made after all options have been fully explained. If the source person is in the high-risk category, or if the source person is unknown, treatment is highly recommended.

Prophylactic treatment involves drinking a specially designed "cocktail" or mixture of drugs. Time counts—the sooner treatment starts, the better. Some sources recommend treatment within two hours of exposure. These drugs are taken at specific intervals for up to four weeks following exposure. This is a rigorous regimen that must be precisely followed. Missing doses could mean developing HIV infection.

These drugs, however, are toxic and unpleasant. Many potentially infected people do not complete the regimen properly because of the side effects. These may include overwhelming nausea and diarrhea, abdominal pain, muscle pain, anemia, neutropenia (the lowering of white blood cells), pancreatitis, altered liver function, and kidney stones. Thus, deciding whether to take the treatment is difficult. For this reason, formal consent for treatment is usually required, and the exposed person is counselled about the risks of the drugs compared with the risks of infection in the particular circumstances. Consent should be obtained from any client undergoing this treatment. Check with your public health unit about regulations in your region.

Follow-up HIV testing is done at regular intervals, usually six weeks, 12 weeks, and six months. Sensitization may not be readily noted. Seroconversion will most likely occur within six to 12 weeks of the event. This is a stressful time for the contaminated person, who should be offered counselling.

Remember the importance of prevention. Ensure that you and everyone else in your workplace have the proper training regarding Standard Precautions, and always follow guidelines to prevent exposure.

DIAGNOSIS If you have a client in your practice who must be tested for HIV, it is important for the physician to explain fully what tests are available, how reliable they are, and how long it will take to get the results.

A common screening test is the enzyme-linked immunosorbent assay (ELISA). This test confirms the presence of antibodies that have developed in response to HIV infection. This test gives false positives approximately 15 percent of the time; so, positive test results are validated with another test known as the western blot test.

TREATMENT OF HIV INFECTION At this point in time, there is no cure for HIV infection, only measures to control the disease. Such drugs as AZT (Zidovudine) boost the function of the immune system in most infected persons. Various "cocktails" are available that help HIV-infected people delay the onset of full-blown AIDS and help those with AIDS live longer. However, these medications have severe side effects and are also very expensive.

INTERACTING WITH HIV-POSITIVE CLIENTS Some health professionals are uncomfortable interacting with people with HIV, let alone having physical contact. Knowledge

POSTEXPOSURE PROPHYLAXIS (PEP) treatment after exposure to a pathogen, aimed at preventing infection.

may counteract fear. Remember that you cannot contract AIDS from casual, everyday contact such as shaking hands or simple touching. Normally, you run no risk in, for example, assisting a client to prepare for an examination or taking blood pressure and vital signs.

Moral judgments and social stigma have also affected attitudes toward AIDS. You must be comfortable interacting with the client as a person before you can be comfortable interacting professionally. Remember that, like all your clients, individuals with HIV or AIDS are people first, not a disease-carrying entity. They are coping not only with a frightening, potentially fatal disease, but often with ostracism by friends and acquaintances. The best thing you can do for someone with either of these diagnoses is to treat them with respect, warmth, empathy, and acceptance.

Preventing Injury in the Health Office

To keep your clients safe, you need to make sure that the physical arrangement of the office is safe and also to plan safe practices, such as ensuring that children are properly supervised. The first step is to understand factors that put people at special risk.

Personal Risk Factors

Childhood

Every growth and development stage has certain typical characteristics. Understanding these patterns will help alert you to potential dangers.

INFANTS Infants are helpless and depend on others to meet all of their needs, including safety. They are curious, like to explore their environment, and have no concept of danger. Infants love to touch and taste; they will grab anything they can reach and put it in their mouth. They are at risk of aspirating foreign objects, poisoning, and falling.

- ◆ If you are weighing a baby, do not take your eyes off her. Even turning your back for a second can result in a fall.
- ◆ Never leave an infant unattended, even in an infant seat.
- ◆ If you notice a parent or caregiver turning her attention away from the baby, for example, when the baby is on the examination table, gently remind her of the dangers.
- ◆ Keep dangerous objects out of the baby's reach. An object is dangerous if it is
  - small enough to swallow,
  - sharp or pointed, or
  - toxic.

(Keep paper out of the baby's reach, too. It probably will not harm the baby, but it will do the paper no good.)

YOUNG CHILDREN As children learn to stand and walk, they greatly increase their mobility. But their sense of danger lags behind. They are curious and imitative and enjoy navigating new environments, including open doors and stairways. Their ability to climb puts them at risk of falling, and increasing problem-solving skills allow them to reach places you might have thought were secure. They love to investigate drawers and cupboards and will often find dangerous objects. Many will still put anything in their mouth, leading to choking or poisoning. They like to mimic others; for example, a child may find a soiled needle and use it to imitate the doctor.

Never allow a young child (under the age of eight) to be in an examination room alone. Watch the child who can open doors and wander off. Keep the lower shelves in the examination room locked or free of anything that might cause injury to a child, such as instruments, sharp objects, and things that can be ingested. Be alert for chairs that the child might climb on to reach a counter, shelf, or examination bed.

If the parent is with the doctor, someone should be available to watch the child either in the examination room or in the reception area. All too often, a parent will leave a child in the reception area, feeling that he is safe because he is occupied with a toy or a book. But children are mercurial, and when the toy loses their interest, they may take up something more dangerous. It only takes a moment for an injury to occur. Normally, you will not have time to assume the responsibility of watching a child.

All toys in the reception area or examination room should meet provincial safety standards and should be safe for children under three.

School-aged children are more aware of danger but, depending on their age and upbringing, often lack the knowledge and awareness to meet all of their own safety needs. Their increased motor skills put more objects within their reach; however, they are increasingly receptive to explanations of danger. Keep in mind, however, that children with developmental delays may be at increased risk.

Visual and Hearing Impairment

Elderly people are particularly prone to diminishing vision and hearing, but these difficulties can occur at any age. Do not assume that only elderly clients suffer from these impairments. Often, people will underplay their disabilities, putting themselves at risk of injury.

Mobility Impairment

Mobility difficulties can range from the most obvious to the subtlest of impairments. The client may, for the most part, manage well and independently. Sometimes anxiety or a current health problem can turn a normally manageable impairment into a problem. Be especially alert for clients with impaired balance, weakness, or an unsteady gait.

Any client who has had a procedure requiring sedation should be assessed for the ability to navigate independently. Sedation may leave clients with slower reflexes such that they are unable to move quickly to avoid injury. Pre-existing mobility problems increase the risk. For procedures requiring sedation, always suggest the client bring along a family member or friend.

Altered Cognition

Some elderly, ill, or developmentally delayed clients may tend to be confused. What may normally be only mild confusion may be compounded by anxiety and stress in the health office. Whatever the cause, confused or very anxious people may not take in information properly or may misinterpret instructions. They may have poor judgment and fail to recognize danger. For example, a client may forget an assistive device and fall.

Fatigue

When people are overtired, accidents happen. People lose dexterity and agility and are more likely to drop things or stumble. Clients may misunderstand instructions or take the wrong medication.

It is not only clients who can become overtired. Try to show up at work rested. If you are tired, be doubly careful about handling sharp, heavy, or delicate objects, and double-check your work. If you sense that you are reaching the point where you can no longer work reliably, tell your employer. It is not heroic to keep working through your fatigue if you make a potentially dangerous mistake, such as handing someone the wrong medicine or dropping a sharp into the wrong container.

Overconfidence

Some people, particularly elderly people with recent impairments, think they can do more than they really can. For example, a person with impaired balance might insist on walking out to the taxi or car without assistance. An understanding, tactful offer of help may be easily accepted.

Environmental Risk Factors

You will be largely responsible for maintaining a safe environment in the health office and reception area. Make sure the environment meets the needs of your specific clients; a pediatrician's office will have different safety needs than a gerontologist's. Be continually alert for areas you can improve upon. Listen to clients' complaints or suggestions.

Lighting

Dim lights in the reception area and halls may predispose clients to falls. Find a balance between dimness and bright, glaring lights.

Noise Level

Children and teens do not appear to mind a noisy environment, but loud noise may be irritating and distracting to adults and may hurt older people's ears or interfere with hearing aids. It may also reduce their ability to concentrate or to understand instructions. If you play music, keep it quiet enough so that people can be heard clearly without raising their voices.

Providing a Safe Environment

- Keep the floors clean and dry, especially during rainy or winter weather. It is fine to post a sign asking clients to remove their boots—but few will. No one wants to remove their boots to walk on a cold and perhaps wet or damp floor. Older people are at increased risk of falling because of mobility problems, poor balance, slower reflexes, and osteoporosis.
- If spills occur, clean them up without delay.
- Pay extra attention to clients with altered vision or mobility problems.
- Periodically check the reception area for scattered books, magazines, and toys.
- Avoid loose scatter rugs. Clients can easily slip and fall or trip over the edges. If you must have an area rug, have a smaller one that fits under a coffee table or some other heavy, fixed structure.
- Arrange furniture, such as coffee tables, out of the way of traffic.
- Do not rearrange the room too often. The unfamiliar layout can be a barrier to clients with poor vision.

Protecting Yourself from Injury

Back Care and Injury Prevention

You may think of back injuries as a hazard of industrial work, but back injuries are common among office workers. It does not always take a huge strain, like lifting a heavy machine, to injure one's back; seemingly small things, like reaching for something from the wrong angle or slumping in front of the computer, can be just as damaging if these actions are repeated daily. Good posture and body mechanics reduce strain on the muscles, joints, bones, and ligaments of the spine.

Key Terms

ACTIVE IMMUNITY 102
ACTIVE INFECTION 97
ACUTE INFECTION 96
AEROBIC BACTERIA 98
ANAEROBIC BACTERIA 98
ANTIBODY 102
ANTIGEN 101
ANTIGEN–ANTIBODY RESPONSE 102
ANTISEPSIS 96
ANTISEPTIC 112
ASEPSIS 107
ASYMPTOMATIC 97
ATTENUATED ORGANISM 102
AUTOCLAVE 114
BACTERICIDAL 112
BACTERIOSTATIC 112
CARCINOGENICITY 93
CHRONIC INFECTION 96
CONTAGIOUS (COMMUNICABLE) DISEASE 96

CONTAMINATION 109
DISINFECTANT 111
DISINFECTION 110
EXACERBATION 97
IMMUNITY 102
IMMUNOGLOBULIN 120
INFECTION 95
IODOPHOR 111
LATENT INFECTION 97
LEUKOCYTES 102
LOCAL INFECTION 96
LYMPH 102
LYMPHATIC SYSTEM 102
LYMPHOCYTE 102
MICROORGANISM 96
MUTAGENICITY 93
NONPATHOGENIC 98
NOSOCOMIAL INFECTION 97
OPPORTUNISTIC INFECTION 97
OTITIS MEDIA 96

PASSIVE IMMUNITY 103
PATHOGEN 97
PHAGOCYTOSIS 102
POSTEXPOSURE PROPHYLAXIS 121
QUALITY ASSURANCE 87
QUARANTINE 108
RECURRENT INFECTION 97
RELAPSE 97
REMISSION 97
SANITIZATION 110
SANITIZER 110
SHARP 111
STERILANT 113
STERILE TECHNIQUE 110
STERILE 110
STERILIZATION 110
SYSTEMIC INFECTION 96
TERATOGENIC 107
TOPICAL 96
VIRULENCE 97

Review Questions

1. What is meant by quality medical care?
2. Discuss the relevance of quality assurance in the health office.
3. What is the purpose of an incident report, and who would initiate it in any given situation?
4. WHMIS lists certain employee responsibilities. Identify and discuss four of them.
5. Draw a diagram illustrating the chain of infection, and explain each step.
6. Describe how the health office professional should deal with used needles, soiled linen, and dirty surgical instruments.
7. Compare and contrast active and passive immunity.
8. What is a nosocomial infection?
9. Explain the different levels of disinfection.
10. In what circumstances should you wear gloves?
11. What should you do if you have been exposed to an infection such as HIV?
12. Why are small children at risk of injury? How can you reduce the risk in your office?
13. What is a cumulative trauma disorder?

Application Exercises

1. In small groups, list and discuss all the things you think are important for a high-quality general practice. Consider both clients' and professionals' perspectives in the office. On the basis of your discussions, draw up a quality assurance manual for the office.

2. Research the policies and regulations for Occupational Health and Safety in your region. If someone in your workplace is injured, how should you care for the injured person and document and report the incident? What are your rights as an employee in your health-care environment?

3. Visit a health-care setting of your choice. (Alternatively, your professor may divide the class into groups and assign a variety of settings.) Prepare by researching the basic elements of WHMIS so that you know what to look for. Find out what materials in each setting are under WHMIS guidelines. How are staff informed about WHMIS? Where do they keep their Material Safety Data Sheets (MSDS) sheets? (If a visit to an occupational setting is not possible, see what you can find by doing an Internet search on the setting of your choice.)

4. Develop an infection control plan for a medical office.

5. You are the administrative manager in a large family practice clinic with four administrative assistants. Hanna, one of the administrative assistants, tells you that Jennifer, another administrative assistant, has confided that she may be HIV positive. Hanna is upset; she does not feel safe working with Jennifer and feels she poses a threat to clients. She challenges you to "do something" or she will. Think of ways that you might effectively handle this situation. State your rationale for each action plan you propose.

6. In small groups, choose a health office setting (dental, optometrist, urgent care centre, family physician). Visit one or more offices (perhaps your own physician or dentist), noting the layout of the reception and office areas. Now design an ideal office, specifying layout and types of furniture. Take into account safety from injury, fire safety, employees' comfort, and safety from cumulative stress injury.

Web Sites of Interest

ISO (International Organization for Standardization) homepage
http://www.iso.org/iso/en/ISOOnline.frontpage

WHMIS overview
http://www.hc-sc.gc.ca/ehp/ehd/psb/whmis.htm

An online course on WHMIS
http://www.whmis.net/

The Canadian Centre for Occupational Health and Safety
http://www.ccohs.ca/

Canada's National Occupational Health and Safety web site
http://www.canoshweb.org/en/

Workers' Compensation Board of Alberta
http://www.wcb.ab.ca/

Workers' Compensation Board of B.C.
http://www.worksafebc.com/

Manitoba Labour, Workplace Safety, and Health Division
http://www.gov.mb.ca/labour/safety/index.html

New Brunswick Workplace Health, Safety and Compensation Commission
http://www.whscc.nb.ca/english/services/
    services.htm

Newfoundland and Labrador Workplace Health, Safety, and Compensation Commission
http://www.whscc.nf.ca/

Workers' Compensation Board of the Northwest Territories and Nunavut
http://www.wcb.nt.ca/

Nova Scotia Department of Environment and Labour (WCB)
http://www.gov.ns.ca/enla/

Ontario Workplace Safety and Insurance Board
http://www.wsib.on.ca/wsib/wsibsite.nsf/public/
    Home_

WSIB Physician Schedule
http://www.wsib.on.ca/wsib/wsibsite.nsf/
    LookupFiles/DownloadableHealth
    ProfessionalFees2001NELAssessment/$File/
    NEL.pdf

Prince Edward Island Workers' Compensation Board
http://www.wcb.pe.ca/

Commission de la Santé et de la securité du travail (Quebec)
http://www.csst.qc.ca/

Saskatchewan Labour, Occupational Health and Safety WCB
http://www.labour.gov.sk.ca/safety/INDEX.HTM

WCB contact information for across Canada
http://www.ccohs.ca/oshanswers/information/
wcb_canada.html

Health Canada, TB Prevention and Control
http://www.hc-sc.gc.ca/pphb-dgspsp/
    tbpc-latb/index.html

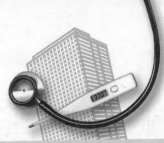

CHAPTER 6
Diagnostic Tests

This chapter gives an overview of diagnostic testing and highlights common tests. The purpose is to make you aware of the more commonly ordered tests and of your related responsibilities. Detailed information can be obtained from any laboratory and diagnostic manual. Specific tests are also discussed in context throughout this book.

LEARNING OBJECTIVES

On completing this chapter, you will be able to:

1. Describe the role of diagnostic tests in client care.
2. Identify the departments of a laboratory, and list the tests associated with each.
3. Discuss the responsibilities of the health office professional with respect to diagnostic tests and procedures.
4. Demonstrate how to fill in requisitions with the required information.
5. Educate clients about laboratory and diagnostic tests.
6. Discuss how to receive and organize test results in the office and hospital settings.
7. Explain how to deal with abnormal results.

Purpose

Medical practice is based on information gathered from a variety of sources, including client history and physical examinations. Diagnostic testing done by laboratory and diagnostic imaging departments provides another valuable source of information to establish a diagnosis and monitor a client's progress and response to treatment. Tests can visualize and analyze body structures, tissues, and fluids. Tests are an important part of health promotion and disease prevention in that they screen for disease, detect problems early, and facilitate prompt treatment. Diagnostic testing can also be used to establish baseline results for clients undergoing treatment or surgery. It may also be used for legal purposes. Results of lab tests are interpreted by a physician in the context of the client's clinical examination and history. The results may validate or invalidate an initial diagnosis; they may lead the doctor to adjust or change the client's treatment plan; they may provide the welcome information that the client is healthy.

A healthy body is said to be in a state of homeostasis, equilibrium, or balance. Each part of the body that is analyzed or examined has what is called a normal range, or a **reference range**. Results of tests are compared with this range. If they fall above or below this range, further investigation is often warranted. Various abnormal tests may, together with a physical examination and client history, lead to a diagnosis. Tests may be ordered individually or as groups, sometimes referred to as test profiles.

Different laboratories may use different reference ranges depending on the analysis type, reagents used, and client population. Thus, the normal ranges presented in this

REFERENCE RANGE the normal range; the values expected for a particular test.

chapter may not be exactly the same as those used at any given laboratory. Always assess any lab result in the context of that laboratory's normal range.

All laboratories should provide normal ranges with test results and flag abnormal results.

Testing Facilities

Diagnostic testing is done in licensed clinical laboratories and diagnostic imaging facilities, both private and within hospitals. A limited number of tests are performed in physicians' offices.

Private laboratories are widespread in Canada. They may be centrally located, with satellite labs in medical buildings, or large ambulatory/urgent care clinics. These facilities offer clinical laboratory services, including routine testing on blood and other body fluids and tissue analysis. Smaller satellite labs in some provinces are referred to as specimen collection labs, and they simply collect specimens (e.g., blood, urine, stool, sputum) and send them to a central laboratory for analysis. Both private and hospital-based diagnostic imaging facilities offer such services as X-rays, **computed tomography (CT)** scanning, **magnetic resonance imaging (MRI)**, **ultrasonography**, and **mammography**. Diagnostic imaging provides a detailed view of structures beneath the skin. Continuing and rapid technological advances in this field have added to its versatility, diagnostic capabilities, and complexity. Advances in diagnostic medicine have contributed significantly to the rising cost of health care in Canada, resulting in long waits for many of these tests.

Canada has national and provincial laboratories that provide specialized services. For example, the National Microbiology Laboratory in Winnipeg conducts tests to diagnose cases of West Nile virus infection. This lab is one of 15 centres worldwide equipped with facilities to deal with biosafety issues, including the most deadly infectious organisms. It is a facility where scientists and researchers can share and discuss information as they study established, emerging, and re-emerging diseases in both human and animal populations.

In most provinces, hospitals have clinical laboratories and diagnostic imaging services. The larger the hospital, the more complex and varied are the testing services it offers. Hospital facilities serve inpatients, outpatients, and the general public. An average-sized hospital typically offers the following laboratory departments:

- Hematology
- Blood bank or blood transfusions
- Chemistry
- Microbiology
- Histology/Pathology/Cytology

Larger hospitals also offer the most complete range of diagnostic imaging services. An average-sized hospital would likely offer the following radiographic studies:

- Routine/plain film X-rays
- Contrast techniques
- Fluoroscopy
- Computed tomography (CT)
- Magnetic resonance imaging (MRI)
- Ultrasonography

Cardiac and respiratory diagnostic services are also offered primarily by hospitals.

COMPUTED TOMOGRAPHY (CT) a type of X-ray that produces three-dimensional images of cross-sections of body parts.

MAGNETIC RESONANCE IMAGING (MRI) a diagnostic tool that uses a magnetic field to produce images of body structures and organs.

ULTRASONOGRAPHY a procedure that uses high-frequency sound waves directed at an organ or object to produce a visual image.

MAMMOGRAPHY a specialized X-ray of the breast.

specific instructions. Many offices use disposable specimen kits that include these instructions. To obtain a midstream urine specimen, the client must carefully wipe the area around the urethra with a cleansing solution. The solution used varies; often, washing with just soap and water is recommended. The client must start to void into the toilet, then stop and collect the middle part of the urine in a sterile container. Most people find it nearly impossible to void into a small bottle; so, many kits supply a larger sterile container in which the person can catch the middle part of the urine stream. This is then emptied into the sterile bottle, taking care not to contaminate the urine or the container edges, and the lid is applied.

Urine specimens for C&S must be taken to the lab immediately or refrigerated. If a specimen sits at room temperature, bacterial growth will interfere with the accuracy of test results. The lab will reject a specimen that has not been handled properly. Remind clients to refrigerate specimens taken at home until they can take them to the lab.

Blood Cultures

Cultures done on blood are ordered if a client is suspected of having septicemia, a blood infection. Infection can spread from various organs or result from surgery. Particularly dangerous is a condition called endocarditis, an inflammation and infection of the lining of the heart and/or heart valves. Although this infection is not common, people who have prosthetic heart valves or prosthetic joints are at increased risk. Blood cultures might be ordered on a client (in or out of hospital) with the onset of a high and otherwise unexplained fever. These are often ordered in groups of two or three to ensure the accuracy of the tests. They may be collected all at once or at designated intervals.

Stool Culture and Analysis

A stool culture and analysis is done to diagnose certain conditions affecting the digestive tract, including infection, poor absorption, or cancer. Lab analysis includes microscopic analysis and chemical and microbiological tests for such organisms as bacteria, fungi, parasites, and yeast. Other elements, such as mucus and blood, are also identified. A common test is stool analysis for occult blood (OB). Stool specimens are often ordered in groups of three, which would be separate samples, perhaps one each day. It

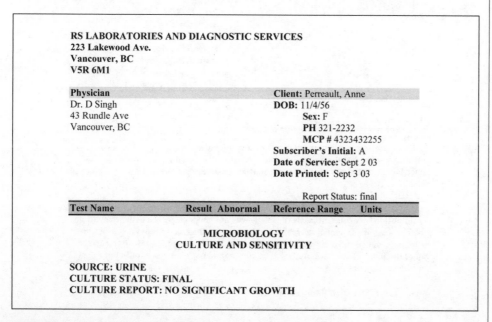

Figure 6.4   Normal urinalysis report for culture and sensitivity.

is sometimes difficult to keep track of specimens obtained in the hospital; so, the nurses usually note when they have obtained a specimen on the client's electronic or traditional kardex (discussed in Chapter 19). Most facilities provide disposable kits for clients to obtain stool specimens. Depending on the test, patients may be instructed to collect the sample in a container, scoop a small portion into a vial, or smear a small amount on special test paper.

Diagnostic Imaging

What was once the X-ray Department in most facilities is now called the Diagnostic Imaging Department because X-rays are only one of the imaging tools available. Newer imaging techniques include computed tomography (CT), magnetic resonance imaging (MRI), and ultrasonography.

X-Ray

A X-ray is a visual test in which an image of a selected body part or region is created by using low doses of radiation reflected on film or fluorescent screens. X-rays can be used to diagnose a wide range of conditions, from pneumonia to a fractured bone. Common X-ray tests include chest X-rays, often ordered as "chest X-ray PA and lateral." This means the doctor wants a front and side view. (See Figure 6.5 for a normal chest X-ray report.) An X-ray can be done on almost any body part, for example, the abdomen, to evaluate trauma or a blockage of the bowel, or the bones, to assess for fractures. Most X-rays require little or no preparation, but you will likely have to book

---

RS LABORATORIES AND DIAGNOSTIC SERVICES
223 Lakewood Ave.
Vancouver, BC
V5R 6M1
Diagnostic Imaging Dept.

Physician	**Client:** Perreault, Anne
Dr. D Singh	**DOB:** 11/4/56
43 Rundle Ave	**Sex:** F
Vancouver, BC	**PH** 321-2232
	MCP # 4323432255
	Subscriber's Initial: A
	Date of Service: Sept 2 03
	Date Printed: Sept 3 03

Report Status: final

Examination Required

CHEST X-RAY – bilateral

The inspiration was suboptimal. The heart is not enlarged. The C/T Ratio is 15.5/26 cm, with a suboptimal inspiration. There is a 1 cm calcified granuloma in the left lower lobe. The lungs and the pleural spaces are otherwise clear.

U/S ABDOMEN

Examination was suboptimal as the client was not cooperative. Grossly, the gall bladder, liver, proximal abdominal aorta, interior vena cava, kidneys, spleen and head and body of the pancreas are unremarkable. Distal abdominal aorta and the tail of the pancreas are not imaged. The common hepatic duct is not dilated, measuring 5.9 cm in caliber.

V.ss   Y.J. Henry MD, Radiologist.

Figure 6.5   Report of a chest X-ray and an abdominal ultrasound.

an appointment for a client to have one done. (See Chapter 9 for booking procedures.) In the hospital, if a client is acutely ill or cannot be moved, the doctor may order a "portable," or you may request a "portable" if the nurses deem it best for the client. The technologist will come to the client's room with a portable X-ray unit.

Endoscopic Retrograde Cholangiopancreatography (ERCP)

An ERCP is a test that uses an endoscope to visualize the liver, and pancreatic ducts. The client is required to remain NPO for eight hours before the test. Because a contrast dye is used, it is important to ask the client about related allergies. Many contrast dyes contain iodine, and so a history of allergies to iodine or past dye tests would be important. Clients find this test very uncomfortable. Despite a local anesthetic, and often an intravenous relaxant, gagging, nausea, and vomiting may occur when the endoscope is passed down the throat.

Barium Swallow

A barium swallow is an X-ray of the throat and esophagus visualized using a contrast medium that is ingested as a drink with the consistency of a milkshake. The passage of the barium through the esophagus and stomach is monitored on the fluoroscope. Pictures are taken with the client in different positions to maximize the view of the GI tract. The test takes 30 minutes to one hour to complete. Similar tests may be ordered as a GI or upper GI series, which focus more attention to the stomach and duodenum.

The client must be instructed to remain NPO for eight hours prior to the test and may be placed on a restricted diet for two or three days prior. It is very important for the client to follow these instructions. Even swallowing a pill may interfere with the examination.

Clients must be advised to take a laxative following the test as the barium can be highly constipating. Let clients know that the first two or three bowel movements may be a greyish-white colour.

Barium Enema

A barium enema visualizes the lower portion of the bowel. Barium is inserted through the rectum prior to the X-rays. The client may be placed on a liquid diet a day or two before the test and may be required to take a laxative the night before. A common one is magnesium citrate, which is very salty. Many clients will tell you that the prep is worse than the test. Those who have experienced it suggest taking the laxative ice cold or sucking on a lemon afterward. If you are booking both a barium enema and a barium swallow for a client, book the barium enema first. If the swallow comes first, the lower bowel may contain residual barium, invalidating or delaying the enema test.

Ultrasonography

Ultrasonography (US), frequently referred to simply as "ultrasound," is an imaging method that uses sound waves with frequencies above detection by the human ear to produce pictures of structures within the body. It is particularly effective in analyzing soft-organ tissue such as the gallbladder, liver, kidneys, ovaries, and bladder. (See Figure 6.5 for an ultrasound report of the abdomen.) Ultrasonography is popular for pregnant women and is the most common investigative procedure in obstetrics and gynecology.

Usually, the HOP will book an appointment for a client's ultrasound. An ultrasound of abdominal organs, particularly for a pelvic examination, may require an empty stomach and a full bladder. The client is instructed to drink about six glasses of water one hour before the test. This fills the bladder, resulting in better visualization of some abdominal structures, especially the uterus. A full bladder is very uncomfortable (whether pregnant or not), and some clients find drinking that much water difficult. Advise the client not to go to the bathroom even if she feels she must. If the bladder is not sufficiently full, the test may be postponed or the client may be asked to drink more water and wait until the bladder is full enough.

CT or CAT Scanning

Computed tomography (CT), also called computerized axial tomography (CAT) or a CAT scan, is a technique using X-rays and a computer to produce cross-sectional images of any part of the body. It often provides more detailed information than conventional X-ray techniques. Common investigations include those of the head, spine, thorax, abdomen, pelvis, and joints. Not every facility has a CT scanner, and so you may need to arrange for a hospital client to have the test done elsewhere.

A contrast dye (that may contain iodine) is used, so allergies must be identified. The part of the body being visualized is positioned inside a cylinder that tilts and rotates to facilitate various views. Claustrophobic people may not be good candidates for this test. The test is, however, less confining than an MRI. Examinations usually take between 20 and 40 minutes. The client may need to arrive an hour early.

Magnetic Resonance Imaging (MRI)

The MRI machine produces a strong magnetic field. When a patient is placed inside this field and the body is exposed to short radio frequency pulses, some of the protons within the cells of the body realign with the external magnetic field. Cells from different parts of the body behave in different ways. Using modern high-speed computers, an analysis of this process can be used to produce images of different parts of the body. MRI is invaluable in diagnosing a wide range of conditions throughout the body and is particularly useful in diagnosing disorders of the brain, spine, and joints.

This test involves moving the client into a tunnel approximately three feet in diameter. Most tests require the client to hold fairly still. Clients who are claustrophobic are poor candidates for an MRI. Clients with metal devices in their bodies are also unable to have an MRI because of the strong magnetic field used for the scan. The doctor needs to know about pacemakers, metal pins or clips, and even tattoos (many contain lead) and IUCDs (intrauterine contraceptive devices). On occasion, a contrast dye may be used, which does not, however, contain iodine. Still, known allergies to any type of dye are important to note.

MRI is not readily available in many communities across Canada. In some regions, the wait for an MRI can be up to a year. If you have a client who is booked several months in advance for an MRI, make a note on your calendar or computer to give the client a reminder call a week or so before the test. Clients forget tests and appointments that are two weeks away, let alone several months. Many MRI machines are operated 24 hours a day to reduce waiting time. If a client does not show up, a resource that could have been used for someone else is wasted.

Mammography

A mammogram is an X-ray of the breast that can be used as a screening mechanism to detect early stage cancer. Most provincial plans will pay for periodic mammograms, usually for older women and those with family histories of breast cancer, who are considered at increased risk. This test must be booked, but waits are usually not long. The test takes about 10 minutes. Many women find the pressure used to compress the breasts painful. Clients may be advised to avoid caffeine for up to two weeks before the test to reduce breast sensitivity. It is also helpful to have the test a week after the client's period when the breasts are less tender. Women having the test for the first time are often quite apprehensive and may ask you if it will hurt. Remember that pain is very

pharmacists are set by provinces but are similar across the country. Pharmacists must graduate from a university program recognized by their governing body and must have practical experience. Provincial regulatory authorities grant pharmacists licences, assess the competency of pharmacists, and ensure public safety. Pharmacists dispense drugs in response to prescriptions written by physicians, dentists, or other designated health providers. They are also an important resource for clients, physicians, and other health professionals. Although most medications are accompanied by explanatory literature, clients often do not understand the sheet or seek more information. Pharmacists will answer their questions, simplify written explanations, and provide more detail as required. Clients may be confused about when to take a medication, whether it will interact with other medications they are taking, and whether there are side effects. Pharmacists can reinforce physicians' information. They will also give advice about OTC drugs and herbal products. Medications are one of the fastest changing components in health care—as fast as some are removed from the market, new ones are approved by the government and introduced to the market.

A pharmacist will review the client's medication profile (based largely on the pharmacy's own records, the client, and information from the doctor) when filling a prescription and will notify the doctor of potential adverse interactions or more effective medications. The pharmacist is often the first to pick up misuse or abuse of prescribed medications and, depending on the situation, will either speak to the client or notify the physician. The pharmacist will advise the physician of new medications, changes in dosage recommendations, and alerts about medications. Pharmacists collaborate with all levels of health professionals to effectively and safely manage clients' medications. They will act as an information resource for you, clarifying medication orders in the hospital and supplementing information in the health office.

Other members of the pharmaceutical team are *pharmacy technicians* and *pharmacy assistants*. Both work under the direction of a pharmacist. Assistants package medication and assist with other dispensary duties and clerical functions. Technicians have greater responsibilities and more extensive training, usually a one- or two-year postsecondary program. They procure supplies, maintain inventories, and help dispense and distribute medications.

Drugs: An Explanation

A drug may be defined as a chemical substance that affects the mind or body, or any chemical compound used to treat or prevent a disease or other condition. In common speech, *drugs* are sometimes thought of as illegal substances, and drugs taken for health reasons are more commonly referred to as *medicines* or *medications*.

Drug Sources

Drugs are derived from a variety of sources.

Plants

Much of the current knowledge about drugs came from herbalists who used plants and herbs in years gone by. They knew through trial and error what herbs, plants, and plant derivatives were effective for various conditions. We use many of their concepts and discoveries in conventional medicine today. Drugs can be obtained from fungi and from the leaves, seeds, sap, stems, fruit, and roots of various plants. The willow tree, for example, contains a component originally used in the production of aspirin. Digitalis is an extract from the leaf of the purple foxglove. Morphine is derived from a gummy substance extracted from the seed pod of the opium poppy. Other products of plants include **fixed oils**, such as castor oil, and **volatile oils**, such as peppermint and clove.

Animal Sources

Animals are a natural source for some medications such as hormones. Originally, insulin was obtained from the pancreas of slaughtered animals, primarily pigs and cattle. Some estrogen is obtained from the urine of pregnant mares. (Synthetic and plant-based forms of estrogen are also available.)

Minerals

Minerals also supply of wide variety of natural drugs, such as potassium and iron supplements, milk of magnesia (a commonly used antacid and laxative derived from magnesium), and lithium carbonate (a salt used to treat bipolar disorder).

Semi-Synthetic

The term synthesis means that something is chemically reproduced. A semi-synthetic drug results when a drug from a natural source is combined with synthetically produced compounds to alter the effect of the medication. The net result of such combinations is a single new chemical formed from some reaction between those ingredients. For example, heroin is a semi-synthetic variant of morphine.

Synthetic

Synthetic drugs are completely formulated in the laboratory. Some are produced using chemicals and others by copying genetic activity in a living organism. Examples of synthetic drugs include diazepam (Valium), ASA (acetylsalicylic acid), ibuprofen, and fluoxetine (Prozac). Synthetic forms of insulin were introduced in 1981. Today, there is widespread use of insulin produced from genetically modified bacteria and yeast.

Drug Names

A single drug can have up to four names. Each refers to the same drug but comes from a slightly different perspective. These names include

- chemical,
- generic,
- trade, and
- botanical.

Chemical

The chemical name of a drug represents its exact formula. For example, the chemical name of bupropion (marketed as Wellbutrin or Zyban) is 1-(3Chlorophenyl)-2-[(1,1-dimethylethyl)amino]-1-propanone. The familiar acetaminophen (Tylenol) is N-(4-hydroxyphenyl) acetanamide. Not surprisingly, these names are seldom used except by pharmacists and manufacturers in the context of chemical interactions and perhaps in research.

Generic

The generic name of the drug is the nonproprietary name given to a medication, or the official name assigned to it. Generic names for new compounds are given out by an

FIXED OILS (also called base or carrier oils) oils, extracted primarily from plants, that do not evaporate.

VOLATILE OILS oils, extracted primarily from plants, that evaporate.

international body to ensure that no two products have the same generic name. The name is much simpler than the chemical name and is not owned by anyone. It does not have protection by copyright. A pharmaceutical company can manufacture a drug (prescription or OTC) under its generic name and put its own trademark on it. Generic names are always spelled in lower-case. Some examples of generic names are

- acetaminophen (one trade name is Tylenol),
- digoxin (trade name Lanoxin), and
- tetracycline (trade name Achromycin V).

Trade name

When a pharmaceutical company develops a new drug, it applies to the government for a patent, which gives it the right to sell the drug without competition for a designated period, usually 20 years. (However, it takes roughly 10 years from the time a pharmaceutical company applies for a patent until the drug is approved for use, reducing the effective patent life of the drug to 10 years.) This system is designed to allow the company to recover its investment in researching and developing the drug and to encourage continued research and development. Most manufacturers select a proprietary (trade) or brand name for a drug once it has been approved for sale. This name receives a registered trademark and is, in most cases, legally protected forever. A brand name may be registered only in certain countries. Anyone can reproduce a drug once the patent has expired but cannot use the original company's trade name. The second company can manufacture the drug under the generic name or can apply for a trademark for a name of its own choosing.

Trade names are always capitalized. Often, the trade names are more familiar than the generic name. People are more likely to have heard of Valium than of diazepam, or of Tylenol than of acetaminophen. However, the use of generic names over trade names is encouraged to avoid confusion.

Generic drugs are generally less expensive than brand-name drugs, partly because the producer of the generic drug is covering only the costs of manufacturing, not of research, development, and extensive advertising. For example, generic acetaminophen is less expensive than Tylenol. Generic ibuprofen is less expensive than Advil, which is the trade name under which one manufacturer produces the same medication. Some companies claim that the trade-name drug is of better quality than a clone with a generic name. Some such claims may be valid because the exact ingredients may differ, resulting in an altered absorption and excretion rate and a slightly different therapeutic effect.

Even when a medication is prescribed by its trade name, the pharmacist can fill the prescription with a less expensive generic form of the medication unless the doctor specifies "no substitution."

Botanical

This is the name used to refer to the natural substance or substances that a drug is made of. An example of this, as previously noted, is *Digitalis purpurea*—herbs from which digitalis is derived.

Drugs and the Law[1]

The regulation and control of drugs in Canada is achieved jointly by the federal and provincial governments. The Health Protection Branch of Health Canada is

---

1. Material for this section contributed by Steve Chapman, author of *Drug Control in Canada*.

chosen pharmacy. If the doctor is seeing another physician's client, an electronic copy of the prescription should be sent to the client's family doctor.

Prescription Forms

Most doctors have prescription forms or pads headed with their name, address, and other necessary information. Figure 7.1 shows the elements of a prescription. Figure 7.2 shows a prescription written in a formal format (for example, with the words "sig" and "mitte" written in); Figure 7.3 shows a prescription written informally, with the names of the elements left out.

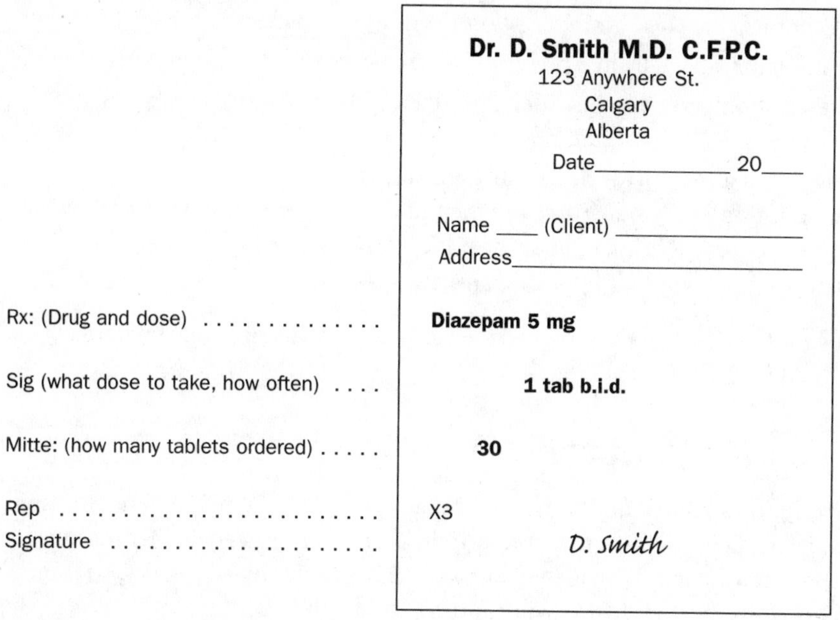

Dr. D. Smith M.D. C.F.P.C.
123 Anywhere St.
Calgary
Alberta
Date_____ 20____

Name _____ (Client) _____
Address_____

Rx: (Drug and dose) . . . .   **Diazepam 5 mg**

Sig (what dose to take, how often) . . . .   **1 tab b.i.d.**

Mitte: (how many tablets ordered) **30**

Rep X3
Signature . . . .   *D. Smith*

Figure 7.1 Parts of a prescription.

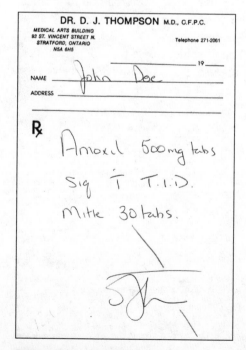

Figure 7.2 A formal prescription.
Courtesy of Dr. Douglas Thompson

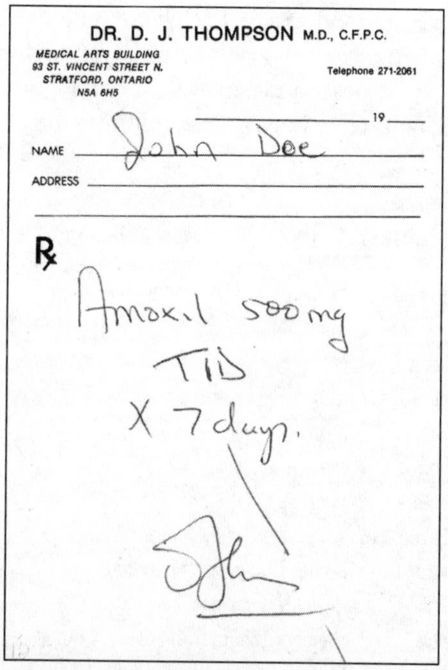

Figure 7.3 An informal prescription.
Courtesy of Dr. Douglas Thompson

Prescription forms must be kept safe because of the danger of theft and forgery, primarily by people who want narcotics, sleeping pills, and tranquilizers.

◆ Keep all prescription pads except for the one in use in a designated locked drawer.

◆ Never leave a prescription pad lying around in your office area.

◆ If you must leave a pad in an examination room, put it out of sight or in a locked drawer.

◆ Ideally, physicians should carry pads in their lab coat pockets.

◆ Never ask the physician to pre-sign a blank prescription.

◆ Do not use the back of prescription forms as notepaper.

◆ If throwing a page from a prescription pad away, shred or otherwise destroy it.

◆ Prescription pads may be ordered tinted to prevent tampering by making erasure or correction fluid obvious.

◆ Suggest that the doctor draw a diagonal line from the bottom of the written prescription to his signature, and then to the bottom of the page, to prevent someone from writing in additional medications.

◆ Prescription pads should be sequentially numbered.

To convey most instructions on prescriptions, doctors use a set of standard abbreviations, listed in Table 7.2.

Repeats and Renewals

Some prescriptions, such as antibiotics, are usually issued for a defined period of time. Once the specified period is over, the prescription is no longer needed. Medications for chronic conditions, such as diabetes, hypothyroidism, or anxiety, may be renewed many times. However, the doctor will want to review the client's condition and the dose from time to time. Prescriptions are often written with a certain number of repeats available (see Figure 7.1). Sometimes, doctors write a prescription for a single period, and either the client calls the doctor's office for a renewal or goes to the pharmacist, who calls or faxes for a renewal.

Repeats and renewals differ slightly, although some people use the terms interchangeably. Repeats are continuations of long-term medications, while renewals are

---

Table 7.2 | Common Abbreviations Used in Medication Orders and Prescriptions

ad lib	as needed by the client	qd	every day (q1d: every day; q2d: every 2 days, etc.)
b.i.d	twice daily		
cap	capsule	q.i.d	four times daily
c̄	with	stat	immediately
gtt.	drop	tab	tablet
hq	every hour	t.i.d	three times daily
h.s.	bedtime	po	by mouth
h.s. p.r.n.	as required at bedtime	IM	intramuscular injection
prn	as necessary, or as required	s.c.	subcutaneous injection
qs	quantity sufficient	IV	intravenously
q. __ h.	every ___ hours (q4h: every 4 hours; q6h: every 6 hours, etc.)	SL	sublingual

extensions of prescriptions that have run out, often one-time or short-term medications. Medications for chronic conditions are usually prescribed with instructions that the prescription can be repeated or refilled a given number of times before a new prescription is necessary. Note in Figure 7.4 that Marlene Blane wants more repeats on her levothyroxine, a hormone replacement she will be on for life. For an example of a renewal, Jorge deSantos was prescribed Voltaren (diclofenac sodium) because his arthritis pain became severe. The doctor thought he might need only one prescription for the flare-up, but when he used up his prescription and went off the Voltaren, the pain became severe again.

Policies for prescription renewals vary with the physician. Many doctors will not renew a prescription over the telephone but insist that the client come in for an assessment. This is prudent because physicians are responsible for any reactions or adverse effects of the medications they prescribe.

When a doctor first writes a prescription, she will include an appropriate number of repeats. When the repeats have been used up, it is time for the client to be seen and reassessed. For example, the doctor may feel it is time to do some blood work on Marlene Blane to see whether her thyroid medication is effective or whether the dose needs to be adjusted. Likewise, birth control pills are routinely prescribed for a year. At the end of that time, the doctor may want to give the client a Pap test and a gynecological examination.

Prescriptions for sleeping pills or tranquilizers will not normally be renewed without an office visit and assessment. You will likely be told to make appointments for clients in such situations.

Some clients resent the inconvenience of having to see the doctor for a prescription renewal. They may feel that it is a money grab on the part of the physician. Actually, the doctor can charge more for a telephone renewal than for a minor assessment.

Most physicians will also refuse to order antibiotics without seeing the client. This is the responsible thing to do. Most often, a swab or other test is done to determine the cause of the infection and to identify the most appropriate antibiotic for the client.

TUESDAY, JANUARY 20TH

Client	Medication	Pharmacy/Comments
Celia Chan wants the following renewed:		
232 Whitlow Cres Kitchener Ph. 231-0000	Valium 5 mg., t.i.d. po Rx # 23443235	Sinclair Pharmacy wants delivered after 5 pm 543-0999
Marlene Blane wants repeats on :		
689 Lake St Waterloo Ph. 543-0000	levothyroxine 0.1 mg po 1 tab q.a.m. Rx# 321 422	Greens Pharmacy husband will pick up after work 232-0000

Clover Pharmacy called wanting renewals for the following scripts:
PH 321-0000
1. Jen Hartlow   digoxin 0 125 mg
2. Jorge deSantos   Voltaren 50 mg, q4h prn
3. Leonard Mihailovic   Wellbutrin SR 150 mg, h.s.

Figure 7.4   Computer-generated list of prescription requests.

Some clients, however, will call stating that they have a sore throat and want an antibiotic to make them better. It is helpful to explain why the doctor wants to see the client before ordering or renewing an antibiotic. As explained in Chapter 5, antibiotics are not effective against viruses. Different antibiotics are also effective against different groups of bacteria. Putting a client on an antibiotic for an infection it cannot cure wastes money and leads to needless side effects. Worse, the bacteria in the patient's body can develop resistance to the antibiotic and can then be passed on to others. The overuse of antibiotics has become a major public health issue as antibiotic resistance increases.

Sometimes, a pharmacy will simply fax the original prescription that the doctor had written when requesting a renewal or repeat, along with a copy of the information put on the bottle at the time the prescription was filled. Figure 7.5 shows a faxed request for a single prescription renewal.

A pharmacist may refuse to fill a prescription because she feels that it is outdated. There are no hard-and-fast rules, but many pharmacists consider prescriptions outdated a year after they are written.

Phoned and Faxed Prescription Requests

In the health office, you will receive many calls about prescriptions from clients, pharmacies, and facilities such as nursing homes. Most will deal with renewals. Physicians will have different protocols on how to manage these calls.

CONFIDENTIAL

COLDWATER PHARMACY
1-222 Lansdowne Ave
Elmira, BC V32 3H4
Ph 613-332-3333

REFILL REQUEST

PATIENT: TANAKA   ALAN
BIRTH DATE: 1966/05/26
PRESCRIPTION NUMBER: 32102222   [Tx 1232222]
LAST REFILL DATE: 24-Aug-03
DRUG NAME: VIOXX 25 mg
GENERIC NAME: ROFECOXIB
QUANTITY DISPENSED: 100 TAB
DAYS SUPPLY: 100

DIRECTIONS FOR USE: TAKE 1 TABLET DAILY

PHYSICIAN: DR.   BROWN   DJ

PHONE: 613-222-2344
FAX 613-443-3333

Number of Refills Authorized	Days between Refills (if applicable)
100	100

PHYSICIAN'S SIGNATURE   DATE

PLEASE FAX BACK TO: 613-243-2333

Figure 7.5 Faxed request for single prescription renewal.

Communicating for Health

CHAPTER8

LEARNING OBJECTIVES

On completing this chapter, you will be able to:

1. Explain the effective use of fax, e-mail, and postal mail.

2. Apply the principles of plain language to the health services setting.

3. Coordinate the use of telephone answering devices and services.

4. Screen, triage, and manage incoming calls.

5. Respond to the individual needs of callers and give appropriate telephone advice.

6. Maintain confidentiality in the health-care setting.

7. Organize and manage outgoing calls efficiently.

8. Respond effectively to difficult and angry clients.

9. Discuss strategies to effectively communicate with health professionals.

Communication in the health office takes many forms. New technologies, such as e-mail, fax, cell phones, pagers, answering devices, and computers, have made communication easier, faster, and more efficient. A doctor can use an Internet link to access a client's test results and X-rays from home or can download client information from a central hospital database before making rounds. Yet, any information exchange system is only as good as the people operating it. The medium of communication is less important than the tone and content of the message.

Excellent communication is critical to good health-care delivery in any setting. Although this chapter focuses on communication in a family physician's office, the same skills and approaches apply whether you work in a specialist's office, a clinic, or a hospital. In the health office, many of the HOP's responsibilities revolve around use of the telephone and other communication devices to collect and relay information, communicate with clients, and coordinate activities. Communication affects client care, treatment plans, appointment scheduling, client education, and interchanges between professionals. Effective health communication is challenging both for clients and for health professionals. Your skill as a communicator is essential not only to make sure everyone gets the information they need, but to make people comfortable.

The Fax Machine

The fax machine is a helpful communication tool. It provides instant relay of information, along with a printed record, and saves phone calls and postal expense. Many offices have a fax/copier combination.

Pharmacies, hospitals, and nursing homes will fax reports, test results, and requests for medication repeats or refills. Physicians will fax requests for consultations and consultation reports. Because a faxed lab report or medication order has all the information in print and need not be transcribed, it saves time and reduces error. The physician can respond to prescription requests right on the fax, which you can then fax back to the pharmacy. Remember, from Chapter 7, that whether a prescription request comes by phone or fax, you must pull the client's chart.

One problem with faxes is that transmissions sometimes get lost. When you receive a fax, check that you have the number of pages noted on the cover sheet. Call the sender if you are missing pages. When you send a fax, specify the number of pages on the cover sheet. Keep a log of all fax transmissions, noting the same information as on the cover sheet. This serves as a record in case a transmission is lost. Most machines will print out a report that the transmission went through, giving date, time, and destination.

A bigger problem with the fax is the risk of breaching confidentiality. Often, fax machines are used by a number of people; some are shared by several offices or hospital departments. It is easy for someone to scoop up a bunch of faxed documents and take someone else's material by mistake. To minimize this risk at your end, try to place your fax machine in a secure area. Watch for expected faxes. When you receive faxed reports, pick them up as soon as you can. Even better, some fax machines come with mailboxes accessible only by code. The sender punches in a code to designate where the fax is being sent. The receiver then punches in the code to activate the printer and receive the message.

E-Mail

E-mail is becoming more popular in health offices and is a useful way to send letters and documents. Some practices make appointments and send clients messages via e-mail. Even if you make all appointments on the phone, it is a good idea to have an e-mail address as another way to contact the client, if you need to.

If you are sending e-mail messages that contain confidential information, you should have security features: encrypt the message, and label the message confidential. Never use a Web-based e-mail service. When receiving e-mail, do not leave anything confidential showing on your screen or accessible to anyone for whom it is not intended.

If you send letters or reports by e-mail, use the same standards as you would for any professional written communication. Use proper spelling, grammar, and capitalization. Too many people have become sloppy with e-mail, treating it as casual conversation. That may be all right for a quick note to a friend, but not for professional messages. When formality is more appropriate, send a properly formatted letter by e-mail attachment.

If you have only one computer in the office, e-mail may not be as convenient. The computer may be needed most of the time for processing health cards, billing, accessing clients' records, and making appointments.

Written Communication

Printed communication in the health office has decreased with the use of the fax machine and e-mail. However, you still need to fill out insurance forms, process return-to-work notes, and perhaps prepare or transcribe consultation reports depending on the type of health office you work in. Many health offices use medical transcription or voice recognition software for creating reports, and then fax them to their destinations.

If you are responsible for typing letters and reports, you need a thorough knowledge of spelling, grammar, and formatting. Reports must be accurately transcribed, professional in language and appearance, and must follow the standard format used at your facility. For the most part, letters will be electronically dictated or, if short, handwritten by the physician. You will likely be expected to edit them for grammar, punctuation, correct word choice, and clarity. Documents created using voice recognition software must be checked for words that were not recognized properly. For example, one report, dictated and sent out unedited, said, "The baby died." It should have read, "The baby cried." It is a good idea to have a letter template on your computer. Most doctors have letterhead stationery.

Some offices send out periodicals updating clients on policies and new treatment options. You may also be responsible for creating client teaching information. Such material must be clear, relatively simple, and organized to make it easy to read. Remember that many laypeople have limited knowledge of medical concepts and terminology. Avoid jargon. If it is simpler to use specialized terms, explain them on first usage.

Signs

If there is something you want all your clients to know, it often makes sense to put a sign in the reception area or at the front desk. For example, you may want to ask clients to call at certain times to schedule appointments (see Figure 8.1). You may want to let them know about office policies, charges for uninsured services, or dates when the office will be closed. You may want to remind them to take off their boots, to show their health cards, or to wait in the office after an allergy injection. The sign needs to convey the message clearly while being appealing and leaving a friendly impression. A few suggestions are:

- Make the sign large enough to be noticed.
- Make the lettering large enough for people with limited vision to read.
- Make the sign simple but attractive. A simple border can help, as can a little colour. Rounded, open fonts are usually more appealing than narrow, heavy ones. Do not use ornate fonts.
- Keep the words brief and to the point.
- Be clear. Ask several people what the sign means to make sure it cannot be misinterpreted.
- Keep a friendly tone. Such phrases as "Please," "Thank you," and "We appreciate," are more courteous than simple commands or words like "must" and "don't."
- Try a little humour. But make sure your wording is not confusing or offensive to anyone.

PLEASE CALL AFTER 10 AM TO MAKE OR CANCEL APPOINTMENTS.

THANK YOU FOR YOUR COOPERATION.

Dr. D. Thompson

Figure 8.1   An office sign.

Incoming Mail

In most offices, mail is delivered daily and arrives either by courier, special delivery, or regular post, which includes priority post and registered mail. You will probably be responsible for sorting and dealing with the mail according to office guidelines. Like phone calls, most incoming mail falls into certain categories.

Medical Reports

Reports may be received on consultations, operations, home care, lab results, and radiology reports. Any lab or diagnostic report must be reviewed and abnormal results flagged for review by the physician. Let the doctor know immediately about abnormal blood sugar and blood coagulation results (e.g., INR, PT, APTT, PTT). Usually, the laboratory will telephone with any critical values; however, never rely entirely on someone else. All reports should be reviewed. Some physicians prefer to do this themselves; others rely on the HOP to review them and to bring abnormal results to their attention. In any case, two pairs of eyes are better than one. Any client with an abnormal result should be notified either by you or the physician, depending on office protocol and the nature of the test.

Insurance Reports

Insurance reports will be sent by private insurance companies, Workers' Compensation Boards, and government agencies. Once the physician completes and signs them, you will send them back. You may have to individualize a reply or attach such documents as medical reports. Where consent is required, do not forget to include the signed form.

Personal Mail

Place any letters or documents marked confidential and any letters you recognize as personal on the physician's desk unopened.

Educational Materials

Educational materials can be for the physician, for the staff, or for clients. If the client-oriented material seems generally useful, you can put it in a rack in the reception area. Some material may be suitable for specific clients only; it can be placed in the examination room or left with the doctor. It is best given out to selected clients as suited. Educational materials for the doctor include a never-ending supply of medical journals, notifications of seminars, updates on drug therapies, and medical newspapers. The physician should sort through these. Replace outdated materials.

Magazines for the Reception Area

Many physicians receive subscription magazines for the reception area. Some of these are promotional and sent free of charge; others may be ordered by the doctor. You may be tempted to "borrow" the magazines that appeal to you. It is fine to read them, but make sure they find their way to the reception area while they are still current. If your physician does not subscribe to any magazines, you might suggest it. The cost of subscriptions can be written off. Reading material in the office should reflect general interests, keeping in mind your client population. For a family doctor's office, cater to various interests with a selection of lifestyle magazines, such as *Canadian Living*, and magazines covering sports, health, travel, science, or culture. For younger clients, include storybooks at various levels. If you work for a gynecologist, you might have a similar selection but with more focus on women's interests. If you work for a pediatrician, you will want more picture books. Have a few board books or washable fabric books for babies.

When conversing with such people, you can feel their warmth and almost see them smile. You look forward to speaking with them. That is what you want to achieve in the health office. If you are one of those natural communicators, you bring a wonderful asset to your job. If not, you can develop your "telephone self" through practice.

- When the phone rings, stop what you are doing to answer the phone. This will help you focus on the call.

- Take a deep breath, and concentrate on the call.

- If someone comes into the office while you are on the telephone, make eye contact, nod, or wave, but remain focused on the caller. When you finish the call, you can attend to the newly arrived client.

- Do not push your mouth up to the mouthpiece of the telephone. This muffles your voice. Have you ever heard someone talk with her mouth on the microphone? A mouth on the mouthpiece produces a similar effect.

- Do not chew gum, eat, or drink when you are speaking on the telephone.

- Smile when you answer the phone, even if you do not feel like it. Some people claim that a smile will make you less tense and more patient and impart a lift to your voice.

- Practise speaking into a tape recorder with various telephone greetings. You might be surprised at how you sound.

- If you have a soft, quiet voice, practise putting more energy into your voice.

- Speak in a lower voice. A lower tone is more soothing and more easily heard and understood.

- Speak more slowly than you usually do. This gives the person at the other end time to take in what you are saying and adjust her thoughts.

- Pronounce each word clearly. Space your words carefully to avoid running them together and sounding garbled.

- Be expressive, avoiding a monotone. This gives interest and meaning to what you are saying and adds appropriate emphasis.

- Do not be embarrassed to use gestures when you are on the telephone; it may enhance the tone and organization of speech. Watch someone talking on the telephone to see how it works. For example, in giving directions, many people will sketch the turns in the air; this helps them sequence what they are trying to explain.

Your choice of words is also important (as it is in face-to-face interactions). Use proper grammar and sentence structure and choose your words appropriately. While proper English usage has relaxed substantially over the last few years, slang and poor grammar have no place in professional conversation. "It don't," "youse guys," "her and I," and "I seen" are some of the errors that will make you sound uneducated and unprofessional. Older people, in particular, will notice this, and in almost every practice today, older people make up a large part of the clientele. If you are not sure about English grammar, take a remedial English course or work through an exercise book. People often fall into error when trying to speak properly. For example, people taught to avoid saying, "Me and Jane are going to the show" may compensate by avoiding "me" entirely, and may end up with sentences like "Please return it to Jane or myself"—which is just as bad.

Sound confident. Avoid muttering "I guess," "I'm not sure," "ummmm," or "I, uh, like, you know." Such vagueness makes the caller wonder whether you are a reliable source of information. If you are asked something that you cannot answer, simply say, "I will have to check that with the doctor," or "I will recheck that policy, Mrs. Rubinoff, and call you right back." You want to convey the idea that if you do not have the information at hand, you know where to get it and will do so promptly.

ANSWERING THE PHONE:
THE SIX P'S

Prompt

Polite

Precise

Professional

Positive

Patient

Answering the Phone

Promptness

Try to answer the telephone before the third ring. This may not always be possible in a busy office, but making a conscious effort will pay off. You may tell yourself that the task you are completing will only take a moment, but it could be seven or eight rings later when you get to the telephone. The caller at this point may be disagreeable and upset, or, worse, it may be an emergency. Usually, it is better to answer the telephone and then get back to what you were doing. *Not* making answering the phone a priority may become a habit that will cause endless irritation in clients.

If you often cannot answer the telephone promptly, you can at least be upbeat about it. Make a bet with the client that you will answer by the fifth ring next time. Even if you do not, you can be sure he will be counting. In most cases, this or a similar technique will lighten the mood.

Greetings

Review the examples below. Which one appeals to you the most? the least?

- "Good morning, Dr. Tremblay's office, Lise speaking."
- "Dr. Tremblay's office, Lise speaking, how may I help you?"
- "Dr. Tremblay's office, Lise speaking."
- "Dr. Tremblay's office."
- "Doctor's office."

Most clients prefer the first, with the second and third ones close behind. The first greeting is complete and courteous. It identifies the doctor's office and the speaker, as do the second and third.

Giving your own name is not only friendly, but helpful. The client may know you by name and feel more comfortable speaking with you. Furthermore, the client may be following up on an earlier phone call or visit and want to speak to the same person as before. Having to explain the reason for the call to someone else is frustrating and could waste your time as well as the client's.

"Doctor's office" is impersonal and lacks warmth. It also does not rule out a wrong number; it could be a different doctor's office. How can you name the doctor if you work for a number of doctors? Some group practices solve this problem with a different line for each doctor. If you have separate lines, answer each with the physician's name. If you have a common line, answer with the name of the group or clinic:

> *"Rankin Medical Centre, Andrew speaking."*

One office manager works for a group of three doctors and answers the telephone simply with "Doctor's office." She claims that this greeting saves time because it is short and direct. But does it? How often does the caller respond, "Is this Dr. Heine's office?" and then, "Is this Diane?" Usually, it saves time to establish identification immediately so that the client can get right to business.

Handling Incoming Calls

Dealing with Volume

You can reduce the number of calls that you receive in the office by asking clients, other professionals, and agencies to fax information, if appropriate. Faxes are particularly useful for prescription renewal requests (see Chapter 7) and test results (see

Chapter 6). A fax gives you a printed copy of the information or request and leaves the phones free for other calls. Some offices are asking that people use e-mail. This is efficient to a point but can become time consuming.

THE MORNING RUSH Be aware of peak times for incoming calls in your office, and make an effort to change some of these patterns. For example, many clients will call for an appointment first thing in the morning. This is likely a busy time for the office staff. You can ask your clients to call for appointments at certain times of the day or post a sign to that effect. (See the discussion of signs earlier in this chapter.)

APPOINTMENT CANCELLATIONS You certainly want clients to call if they have to cancel an appointment. However, to reduce the volume of incoming calls, some health offices have a telecommunications system that asks clients who are calling to cancel or reschedule to leave a message. These messages must be checked at regular intervals.

CLIENTS CALLING FOR CLARIFICATION OF INSTRUCTIONS A common type of call will be from clients seeking information. You can help reduce this type of call by clearly and concisely explaining any instructions to the client about tests and appointments (see Chapter 6). Whenever possible, give out printed instructions. Highlight relevant areas. Avoid medical jargon that might confuse the client. It is worth taking a couple of extra minutes to explain something thoroughly if it saves having to explain it all over again over the phone.

CLIENTS CALLING FOR TEST RESULTS Try reversing the process. Tell clients that you will call them if there is any concern about the test results. If clients want to know either way, tell them you will call with results within a certain time frame. This obviously depends on the type of test; results from simple blood work can be back within 24 hours, while biopsy results may take a week. You could also advise clients to call the office if they have not heard from you by a certain date. This still gives you the opportunity to call, but does not leave the client sweating for weeks if you forget or the test is delayed.

Handling Typical Calls

Most calls in a doctor's office fall into certain defined categories. Your first decision is regarding which calls to handle yourself and which to pass on to the doctor. If there is a nurse, she can take a number of the calls that you would otherwise route to the doctor. The nurse and the doctor should agree just what types of calls the nurse can handle— usually questions about immunizations and other health-related issues. If the nurse takes a call that she feels she cannot handle, she will direct the call to the physician.

Table 8.1 assumes that there is no nurse in the office and divides typical calls into three categories: those that you or another HOP can usually handle, those that should be directed to the doctor (either immediately or as a message to call back), and those that fall into a grey area. The ones in the middle you may be able to handle after consultation with the doctor, or you may be able to handle in part before leaving a message for the doctor. The physician should establish clear policies on how to handle different types of calls.

Drug Representatives

Drug reps are people employed by drug companies to promote their company's line of medications. They visit doctors' offices to discuss their products and sometimes leave samples. The reps may call for an appointment or simply arrive at the office. Most doctors set specific times—perhaps every Friday from 11:30 to 12:00—when they will meet with the rep. You need to know the policy, make sure the drug reps know it, and adhere to it. Encourage reps to call the day before to confirm the appointment. Remember to notify drug reps as well as clients if you have to cancel appointments.

Table 8.1 | Routing Typical Calls

Calls You Can Handle	Calls That You Might Handle with Consultation	Calls to Direct to the Doctor
Drug reps	Clients asking for medical advice	Other doctors wanting to speak to your doctor (Always put through another physician unless specifically advised otherwise.)
Clients calling to make appointments	Clients calling to request the results of lab tests	The hospital wanting orders on a client who has been admitted or asking to change or renew an order
Clients calling for information about family members	Calls relating to prescription renewals/repeats	
Clients wanting to talk to staff members	Clients wanting to speak with the doctor	The hospital calling about a change in a client's status (Always put this through. It may be an emergency.)
Individuals looking for a doctor	Laboratories calling with test results	Community agencies calling to speak with the doctor about clients under their care
Laboratories or diagnostic facilities calling to confirm or change appointment times		Personal calls for the doctor
Hospitals calling with a date for a client's surgery		

Clients Calling to Make Appointments

This type of call is generally straightforward, and the HOP would handle it. The only time you may want to check with the doctor would be if the client had spoken to the doctor with a special request for a visit outside of office hours. Unless the doctor had told you about this, you would confirm with her.

Remember that when clients call to make an appointment, it is for a reason, usually related to a health concern. One cannot overemphasize the importance of a pleasant telephone manner in this situation. Be positive and helpful. Try to accommodate the client's request, but remain in control by offering choices. Never use barrier words such as "I can't," "you can't," "it's impossible." Instead, try the following:

> *"Mr. Li, which would be better for you, morning or afternoon?" I'm sorry Mr. Li, I don't have anything for late morning. I can fit you in on Wednesday at 9. I realize that's somewhat early for you, but the advantage is that you won't have to wait. Later in the morning, on Wednesdays in particular, we get very busy and often run a bit late. Now, I could give you an appointment next Monday morning, but that's 6 days away. Would you prefer that?"*

You are keeping control while offering Mr. Li choices.

Appropriate use of triage is essential. Anyone whose problem sounds urgent should be seen immediately or sent to the Emergency Department. Anything like chest pain, shortness of breath or other breathing difficulties, loss of consciousness, profuse bleeding, loss of function of body parts (for example, inability to effectively move one side of the body), or loss of sensation must be dealt with immediately as should earache, high fever, or UTI. The doctor should provide you with criteria for triage both in the office and over the telephone. Remember that it is not your responsibility to make medical decisions, but you should know how to direct clients with health concerns. You will gain experience at triage, but never second guess a client in distress. When in doubt, err on the side of caution and assume it is an emergency: check with the doctor immediately, and/or send the client to the nearest ER. A needless emergency visit or a little disruption is better than a preventable death or permanent disability.

Clients Asking for Medical Advice

The best advice here is "Don't." An exception is triaging obvious emergencies. Your employer may also define certain areas of knowledge and experience within which you may give advice. For example, if a mother calls asking when to bring her child in for

When the Client Is Leaving

Unless clients have to book an appointment or a test, they often leave without saying goodbye. They may be feeling confused about the instructions they have been given or disturbed about some information the doctor has given them. Acknowledging their departure gives you the opportunity to pick up such cues and respond accordingly, answering questions or offering a comforting comment if appropriate. A smile, "good-bye," "It was nice to see you," or even a wave is good client relations if you can manage it.

Dealing with Difficult Situations

You must be prepared to interact effectively, both in person and on the telephone, with clients in a variety of situations. Inevitably, some clients will be angry, rude, or just plain difficult. They may be upset, anxious, stressed, or confused. How a person reacts will reflect a combination of his personality and the situation he finds himself in.

If not handled sensitively, an angry and upset client may become increasingly louder and sometimes aggressive. Your challenge is to maintain your composure and try to contain the situation. Waiting to see the physician is an ongoing source of irritation in many health offices. Some clients relax with a book, others mutter good-naturedly, and still others become openly resentful. Other issues upset clients as well: a lab test result that they were not notified about, a long wait before they can see a specialist, a mix-up in appointment dates, problems with prescriptions, or unmet expectations of health care. Sometimes, clients' distress about bad news may turn to anger.

Often, anger begets anger. Have you ever come home in a good mood only to find an argument in progress? You probably found your own mood deteriorated quickly. If a family member confronts you angrily, how do you respond? Most people will become defensive and show their own annoyance in word and gesture. But what can this entirely natural reaction lead to? An escalated argument.

Business people often say, "The customer is always right." In a sense, the same principle applies to health care. As discussed in Chapter 1, we no longer deal with *patients* who are expected to passively receive care, but with *clients* who are active consumers of health care. If your practice is client driven, your goal is client satisfaction and retention. Dealing effectively with difficult situations goes a long way toward achieving client satisfaction.

The key to dealing with angry or upset clients is to show genuine warmth, respect, and empathy. If you are taking or have taken a communications course, you will be familiar with these variables. Apply them to health-care situations.

Warmth is difficult to define but makes a world of difference. It can be displayed through words, voice, facial expression, and eye contact. Over the telephone, a soft tone of voice can convey warmth, as can words that express concern for the client. Emphasizing some words can also display warmth.

> *"Mr. Martinez, I am so sorry that you were kept waiting so long."*

Being treated with *respect* is a fundamental human right and is especially important in health care. A client who feels respected will be better able to calm down and deal with issues. One way to show respect is simply to pay full attention as you allow the client to express her thoughts and feelings. If the complaint is long, acknowledge that you are listening with the occasional "uh huh" or "I see." You may also ask for clarification: "Miss Hakimi, I'm not sure I understood that last part . . . would you repeat the part about the X-ray getting lost?" Using the client's name also signals respect for the individual.

Empathy is the ability to put yourself into the client's situation. Understanding where the client is coming from does not have to mean that you agree, but it does give you a deeper appreciation of how the client is feeling. If you can show that you understand where the client is coming from, without judging, the client will feel more accepted and valued. Try such phrases as the following:

> *"I understand how you must be feeling, Mr. Amadou."*
> *"You seem very worried, Ms. Carr. Let's look at the options we can consider here and find out what would be best for you."*

Met with warmth, respect, and empathy, most people have a hard time staying angry. Certainly, their problem does not disappear. However, the level of anger and anxiety may subside, paving the way for meaningful dialogue about solutions.

The Aggressive, Unpleasant Client

Remain calm. Remind yourself that the anger is not aimed at you personally. When people are angry, they often take it out on the nearest person. Separating yourself from the situation helps you keep your emotions in check. Speak as slowly as usual, and do not raise your voice, even if the client is shouting. The last thing you want is a shouting match. A technique that sometimes works is to actually lower your voice. The client will have to stop talking to hear what you are saying.

It is important to retain control of the conversation. Be firm, but do not argue with the client. Do not give the client something more to argue about; stick to the issue at hand. Sometimes, a response such as "I'm so sorry, that sounds like it was very upsetting for you," will take the wind out of the aggressive client's sails. Remember, often the client really does have a valid concern or complaint. If the complaint is justified and the office is at fault, acknowledge it and apologize. Try to find a way to rectify the problem immediately. In some situations, all you can do is apologize. If there is a reasonable explanation for the error, tell that to the client. It will not right the wrong, but it might help her understand why it happened. If there are steps you can take to prevent a similar error from occurring again, assure the client that you will take them.

As discussed in Chapter 2, sometimes the client's perspective may be altered because of illness or an emotional reaction to the illness of a loved one. That does not make the issue any less real for the client. Regardless of the situation, if you make clear to the client that you will work *with* him, you will usually get somewhere.

Ask the client what he sees as a possible solution. People will often calm down when they feel they have input and are listened to. If you have several options to deal with the issue, offer all of them, and ask the client which he thinks is most appropriate. If the issue is something that you cannot rectify, assure the client that you will look into the matter and get back to him with an answer or direct him to someone who can help. Give a time frame. "I understand, Mr. Premsyl. I will talk to Dr. Matthews when she gets in after lunch and call you back before 4 o'clock, if that's convenient for you."

Sometimes, writing down the concerns may help a client calm down and refocus. Assure the client that you will give what he has written to the appropriate person.

If the client is rambling and you cannot get a word in edgewise, try raising your hand into the stop position. The client's eyes will follow your hand, and usually, she will stop talking for a moment. Use this opportunity to interrupt: "Celina, I think I understand what you are saying. Let me rephrase the problem, just to be sure. I don't want to miss any of the facts here." This response requires the client to pay attention to what you are saying and lets the client know that her complaint has been heard and that you are taking steps to deal with it.

Remember, when you were little, how you felt when your mother said *NO!* or *You can't,* or *I won't allow you,* or *Never?* You probably felt backed into a corner and more determined than ever to do whatever you were not allowed to do. To an angry person, these words are like a red flag to a bull. Instead, use conciliatory and nonjudgmental language.

The Threatening Client

If you are facing an angry or aggressive client across your desk, stand up. If you are sitting and the client is standing, that puts the client in a position of power, physically as well as emotionally, and makes you seem more vulnerable.

Rarely, you will face a situation you cannot deal with. It is no shame to admit it. Remember that you matter, too. Patience has its limits; you should not tolerate being abused or threatened.

Some sources will advise you to put a disruptive client into a separate room, such as an empty examination room or the doctor's office. While this might work in some situations, in your particular situation, use your good judgment. If possible, call the doctor out to support you and perhaps take control of the situation. Never enter a room alone with a client who makes you feel threatened. Do not let the client stand between you and the door of the room. If you ever feel that your safety is threatened, tell the client that you are going to call the police. Then, do it.

TIPS FOR DEALING WITH DIFFICULT CLIENTS

> KEEP CALM.

> DO NOT TAKE IT PERSONALLY.

> LISTEN TO THE COMPLAINT WITHOUT INTERRUPTING, AND THEN RESTATE IT.

> USE THE CLIENT'S NAME FROM TIME TO TIME.

> KEEP YOUR VOICE QUIET, EVEN IF THE CLIENT IS SHOUTING. TRY LOWERING YOUR VOICE.

> TRY TO PUT YOURSELF IN THE CLIENT'S SHOES.

> ACKNOWLEDGE THE CLIENT'S ANGER OR FRUSTRATION.

> DO NOT BLAME THE CLIENT.

> ASSURE THE CLIENT THAT YOU WILL DO EVERYTHING YOU CAN TO HELP. OFFER OPTIONS.

> NEVER ARGUE WITH THE CLIENT OR USE PROVOKING WORDS OR PHRASES, SUCH AS *NEVER, CAN'T, WON'T,* OR *YOU'RE MISTAKEN.*

> IF THE COMPLAINT IS JUSTIFIED AND THE OFFICE IS AT FAULT, ACKNOWLEDGE IT AND APOLOGIZE.

> IF THE CLIENT BECOMES VERBALLY ABUSIVE, SWEARS, OR THREATENS, SIMPLY SAY, "MR. LEUNG, I CANNOT HELP YOU IF YOU CONTINUE SPEAKING TO ME LIKE THAT."

> IF A CALLER CONTINUES TO BE ABUSIVE, SAY, "MR. LEUNG, I WILL NOT LISTEN TO THAT KIND OF LANGUAGE. PLEASE CALL BACK LATER. GOODBYE." THEN, HANG UP.

> IF YOU CANNOT RESOLVE AN ISSUE, CONSIDER PASSING IT ON TO THE DOCTOR. SOME CLIENTS FEEL THAT THE DOCTOR IS THE ULTIMATE AUTHORITY AND THAT THEY HAVE WON THE BATTLE BY BEING ABLE TO DISCUSS THE ISSUE WITH THE PHYSICIAN.

> DOCUMENT THE COMPLAINTS ON THE CLIENT'S CHART AS SOON AS POSSIBLE WHILE THE DETAILS ARE FRESH IN YOUR MIND. DO NOT RECORD IMPRESSIONS OR INTANGIBLES. WHENEVER POSSIBLE, USE DIRECT QUOTES.

> TELL THE DOCTOR WHAT OCCURRED. THE DOCTOR MAY NEED TO DEAL WITH THE OCCURRENCE THE NEXT TIME THE CLIENT COMES INTO THE OFFICE. IT IS IMPORTANT TO WORK AS A TEAM. EVEN IF YOU OR THE DOCTOR IS IN THE WRONG, ACKNOWLEDGING THE FACT TOGETHER REINFORCES YOUR OFFICE'S COMMITMENT TO GOOD CLIENT CARE.

The Anxious Client

Skill and patience are also needed in dealing with anxious clients. Speak to them especially warmly and gently. People who are stressed, anxious, and preoccupied with thoughts of, for example, an illness or the prospect of an operation are less able to take in and retain information. This temporary loss of capacity will compound forgetfulness and confusion in anyone (elderly or not) with cognitive impairments. If you see that a client is anxious, carefully explain whatever she needs to know about medications, treatments, and subsequent appointments, and reinforce the information by writing it down.

Know Your Limits

Throughout this section, I have emphasized the need to make the client feel important. But you are important, too. You are human, and you, too, have emotions. There will be times when your own concerns make it very difficult to maintain the calm, warm, unruffled manner you would like. If the problem is work related, try to resolve it promptly. The tension of an unresolved conflict in the office cannot but affect how you relate to others. Approach the person(s) involved, and tactfully address the matter. If you do not feel the parties involved are able to deal with the issue fairly and responsibly, try to get a third party to help resolve the conflict, perhaps the office manager or the doctor.

Personal issues likewise cause strain and undermine your ability to deal with other people and their problems. If possible, deal with personal issues at home, and shelve them while at work. But recognize that this is not always realistic. You are not doing yourself or anyone else any favours if you ignore your personal problems when they adversely affect your performance. You have to balance your own physical and emotional health needs with the demands of your job, even if it means taking time off.

Professional Communication

So far, I have emphasized the importance of communication with clients. It is equally important to communicate effectively with other health professionals. Even within the office, miscommunication can turn an otherwise pleasant workplace into a minefield.

What undermines good communication in the office? Stress, of course, is a factor. However, staff members who have a good working relationship will not take the occasional stress-induced flare-up to heart. Territorialism also leads to trouble when staff members guard their own job responsibilities so jealously that they resent anyone who tries to help. A health-care setting requires a certain amount of sharing. Teamwork is the backbone of any successful enterprise. If you see that a colleague is feeling pressured or overwhelmed, offer to help, if possible; it can make a huge difference.

Each staff member will have a certain level of expertise in a given area. Sometimes people, especially if they are insecure or lack self-confidence, will not ask for help because they do not want to acknowledge that someone else might know more than they do about a particular subject or procedure. Office professionals can end up working alone in the same office, isolated by defensive attitudes and not benefiting from co-operation. It is so much more effective to give each person credit for what she does well and to share knowledge and experience.

Always treat others with respect. Comment positively on what a co-worker does well. If you see someone doing something you think you could do better, assess the situation before you speak. Sometimes it is better to keep quiet. If you feel you must offer advice, do so constructively. Ask for help if you need it. Most of us are pleased to share knowledge with someone who appreciates it.

If you are making an appointment for a new client or someone with whom you are not familiar, try to determine if they have special needs so that you can accommodate them as much as possible. I once made an appointment over the telephone for a client who had never been to the office. She arrived in her wheelchair only to find that the office was not wheelchair accessible. She had to return home without being seen. (The doctor made a house call later in the day.)

Pre-office Conference or Information Update

You may review the day's appointments with the provider, using a day sheet or the appointment book, at the beginning of the day and before the doctor starts seeing clients in the afternoon. Some physicians also like updates midmorning and mid-afternoon. This quick meeting facilitates good communication and helps the day run smoothly. It lets the doctor know what is happening and how heavy the day is and gives both of you the opportunity to talk about other matters. You can ensure that the doctor knows about any activities he is scheduled for that day; he may have forgotten about a commitment made weeks ago. Also, ask if the doctor has anything to add to the schedule; he may have forgotten to tell you about something that came up at the last minute. Doctors have been known to encourage a client to "just drop in this afternoon," which plays havoc with your appointment schedule. You have to deal with these clients, try to fit them in, and often make scheduled clients wait. You need to communicate clearly with the doctor about the problem; you can request that he not do this, except in special circumstances. If he does, he should at least let you know so that you can pull the client's chart and be prepared. If clients are expecting to pick up forms, you can give them to the doctor or remind him to complete them. You can also present any abnormal lab tests to the doctor, receive instructions on dealing with them, and ask any questions you may have about other issues or reports.

Confidentiality and the Appointment Book

The appointment book contains confidential information and must be kept away from the view of others. If possible, keep it away from a door or reception window, and do not put it on a desk at which you interact with clients. If it must be in such a location, keep it closed. At the end of the day, put it in a secure place. Otherwise, it can innocently be seen by the cleaning staff and anyone else with access to the office.

If you are using a computer appointment system, place the monitor at an angle that does not allow clients to read it. Turn the monitor off when you are not using it. Many offices store other client information and files on the computer as well, so limit computer access to appropriate individuals. Keep all passwords confidential and, if written down, stored securely.

The appointment book is a legal document. If you make a mistake or change appointments, do not erase; instead, rule a neat line through the error, and write in above it. An alternative for computerized systems is to note no-shows and cancellations on the daily appointment schedule or day sheet. You should also note this information on the client's chart.

Types of Scheduling

A number of different scheduling methods are currently used in health care. Each has its own advantages and disadvantages and suits some types of practice better than others.

Fixed Office Hours, or Open Scheduling

With this method, the facility is open at certain hours, and clients may come whenever they like within those hours without an appointment. Few family practices use this method, but it is used in some group practices and is the norm in walk-in and urgent care clinics based on the principle of providing care to clients when they need it. Clients first see the HOP, have their health card validated, and explain the purpose of the visit. Clients in urgent need of care are seen first; otherwise, clients are seen in the order in which they arrive. The client must understand that barring an emergency, they will be seen on a first-come basis.

This method eliminates the work of maintaining schedules and the problems of missed or cancelled appointments and late arrivals. It suits some clients with busy and irregular schedules.

One obvious drawback to this method is the unpredictable variations in workload. There may be very slow periods, in which staff time is not used effectively, and times when both you and the doctor are so busy that it is difficult to cope. Another drawback, for a practice, is that you have no time to pull the client's chart ahead of time, no opportunity to validate the health card, and no idea what the presenting problem is. You have no time to prepare for procedures required for particular complaints, such as syringing an ear.

If you are working in a walk-in or urgent care clinic, the client is unlikely to have a chart there. All information is recorded on a facility admission sheet and perhaps a progress, multidisciplinary, or fact sheet. You will take the necessary client information, process the health card, and record the reason for the visit. The physician will record the details of the visit on the appropriate record. Forward duplicates to the client's family physician.

Wave Scheduling

WAVE SCHEDULING booking several clients for the same block of time, typically an hour.

Wave scheduling is a compromise between open scheduling and scheduling by appointment. This method is so named because clients come in groups, like waves hitting a beach. A certain number of clients are booked to see the provider within a given time frame (see Figure 9.7). You might find this type of scheduling in the office of an allergist or an endocrinologist. First, determine how many clients the provider can see in the time frame (see the discussion later in this chapter). For example, if Dr. Meiros usually sees one client every 10 minutes, he will see approximately six clients in one hour. You would then ask six clients to come in between 0900 and 1000 hrs, and another six between 1000 and 1100 hrs. They are not given specific times. The premise is that some clients will come earlier than others. It allows clients some flexibility, while still offering some structure and control. You can pull charts and validate health cards ahead of time. The drawback is that if all the clients in a wave arrive at the same time, some will have to wait longer.

Modified Wave Scheduling

Modified wave scheduling uses a basic block of time, as does wave scheduling. However, clients are given narrower time slots to control traffic flow more closely. For example, you might ask two clients to arrive between 1 p.m. and 1:15 p.m., another two to arrive between 1:15 and 1:30, and so on.

Affinity Scheduling

AFFINITY SCHEDULING (also called CLUSTER, CATEGORIZATION, or ANALOGOUS SCHEDULING) scheduling similar appointments together, for example, scheduling physical examinations on a certain day.

Affinity scheduling, also called **cluster**, **categorization**, or **analogous scheduling**, involves scheduling clients in clusters on the basis of the type of service or reason for

Monday Jan 13	Tuesday Jan 14	Wednesday Jan 15
0900 George Papadakis 321-2222 Alice Leroux 543-4444 Harry Fong 543-4340 Edgar Hewitt 654-5655 Boris Karsch 543-5555 Ginny Trotter 654-6545	**0900** Ryan O'Donnell 654-5665 Maria Andre 654-6545 w 443-4444	**0900** Harriet Reis w 543-4544 Austin Pringle 543-5444 Connor Palmer 654-6666 Tiffany Thompson w 645-4444
1000 Manuel Olveidos 543-5444 w 543-5555 Chris Robb 654-6545 Melanie Chang cell 543-4444 Krista Oran 543-5434 Mattie Brown 543-5446 Sarah Sittlinger 364-9849 1100	**1000** Jack Bonham 555-5555 David Rhys 654-6545 Sam Benito 654-6599 June Gibbons 234-0987 Maurice Loton 956-2538 1100	**1000** Wendy Chee w 543-0987 Susanna Diaz 203-5934 Cecil Kondo 232-9876 Donny Bernier 238-6543 Serena Donnelly w 543-4444 1100

Figure 9.7 A sample appointment book showing wave scheduling.

seeing the doctor. Many dental offices, as well as some medical practices, use this method. For example, the dentist may see clients who need check-ups on Monday and Wednesday mornings and those who require uncomplicated fillings on Tuesday and Thursday afternoons. Monday and Wednesday afternoons may be surgery days, and Fridays reserved for orthodontic procedures. A general surgeon might see all clients with breast lumps on a certain day, those with abdominal complaints another day, those who need follow-up assessments another day, and so on. Primary care physicians do not usually use this method of scheduling exclusively.

Affinity scheduling maximizes the use of special equipment that may be needed for certain procedures and makes it easy to determine how much time to allow for each appointment. However, repetition can become boring for the provider. Furthermore, in a given week, the range of clients' problems may not fit the affinity schedule. This form of scheduling also leaves fewer choices for clients.

Combination or Blended Scheduling

Often, a medical practice will use a mix of randomly scheduled appointments with affinity scheduling to create what is called **combination** or **blended scheduling**. Many physicians will do annual physicals and pre-operative examinations on certain mornings, perhaps Monday and Wednesday mornings. They may see prenatal clients and do well-baby examinations on Tuesday and Thursday mornings. The rest of the time is open for any type of complaint. Individuals who require allergy injections may be asked to come in on Tuesday and Friday afternoons. The doctor must be in the office when a client has an allergy shot in case there is an adverse reaction, but if there is a nurse to give the injection, the doctor does not usually have to see the client. Figure 9.8 shows a schedule that uses affinity scheduling on Monday, Tuesday, and Wednesday mornings. From Wednesday afternoon appointments are random.

Advantages to this type of scheduling include organization and making optimum use of specialized equipment. Annual medicals, for example, take anywhere from 20 to

COMBINATION SCHEDULING or BLENDED SCHEDULING a combination of affinity and random scheduling.

Monday January 10 Prenatal visits am/Well baby pm.	Tuesday Jan 11 Pre-op and Annual CPX	Wednesday Jan 12
9:00 Sally Okson 432-4433	9:00 Doreen Marshall 654-5554	9:00 Marta Skrypec back pain 544-0909
9:15	9:15	9:15 John Stouffer BP check 388-7926
9:30 Eliz McVey 543-444	9:30	9:30
9:45	9:45 Anil DaSilva 432-3543	9:45
10:00	10:00	10:00 Peter Chong sore throat 365-3552
10:15	10:15	10:15 Ahmed Kassam, knee pain 548-8320
10:30	10:30 Courtney Edwards	10:30
10:45	10:45 543-5543	10:45
11:00	11:00	11:00
11:15	11:15	11:15
11:30	11:30	11:30
11:45	11:45	11:45
12:00	12:00	12:00
1:00 Brandon Spears 432-3333 bronchitis	1:00 Val McPherson 432-3543	1:00 Bo Keen earache 432-3333
1:15 Ben Hanson 432-3333 abd pain	1:15	1:15 Sharon Dewey rash 543-4444
1:30 Kayleigh Meyers 432-4443 sore throat	1:30 Alicia Torres 984-4444 leg pain	1:30 Patti Haines follow-up burn 543-8654

Figure 9.8   An appointment book showing a blend of affinity and random scheduling.

30 minutes. Doing them on specific days allows the rest of the week to be used more efficiently for more routine encounters and avoids delays caused by lengthy appointments. Booking an annual examination in the middle of a busy afternoon when the reception area is full and you are already running 45 minutes late will only add to the stress for you and the waiting clients.

Assess the scheduling pattern in your practice. You may be able to introduce some changes that enhance efficiency.

Double, or Double-Column, Booking

DOUBLE BOOKING or DOUBLE-COLUMN BOOKING booking two client appointments at the same time, on the assumption that one of the appointments will involve little of the doctor's time.

Double booking is rarely used as the *primary* scheduling method in any facility. However, when a busy office or clinic already has a full schedule and has to accommodate emergencies, double booking can lend a semblance of order to what could be a booking nightmare. The additional clients' names are entered into a second column or row, beside or underneath the names of the regularly scheduled clients (see Figure 9.9). On

Time	Client	Ph#	Comments	Client
1300	Marysia Lovic	432-3432	Well baby	Amanda Kloff/allergy shot # H421-9420
1310	Allyson Baker	232-3232	Prenatal	
1320	Michael Liu	543-5434	Earache	Dana Black/rash # 222-1110
1330	Greg Ivanovich	543-5434	Fatigue	
1340	Lillian Atkins	543-4543	Follow up ear infection	Simone Garlinsky/suture removed # 469-2197

Figure 9.9   An appointment book showing double booking.

Booking Appointments for Tests

Physicians often order procedures or laboratory tests for clients. All tests require a requisition, as discussed in Chapter 6.

Blood Work

Routine blood work does not usually require an appointment. However, the client may need directions to the laboratory and the hours of operation. The client may have a choice of laboratories, which may be in-hospital or private facilities. If your office is in a medical building, you may have a laboratory on site (sometimes called a bleeding station, or satellite lab). Provincial insurance usually covers the cost of tests at any lab. The client can choose whichever is more convenient. Usually, clients are given the requisition to take with them to the lab. Some practices fax the requisition directly to the lab.

Diagnostic Tests

Diagnostic tests are more likely to require appointment times, and some require special preparation (see Chapter 6). Before booking the appointment, ask the client for a range of convenient days and times. The exception is for such tests as MRIs, which, in some parts of the country, currently have waiting periods of up to a year for nonurgent cases. In this case, take whatever appointment you are offered. Once the appointment is made, give the client written verification of the date and time. Send or fax the requisition to the appropriate facility. Some practices may give the requisition to the client to take with them. However, if the client loses or forgets the requisition, the procedure may be delayed or cancelled.

Booking Clients for Surgery

Often, a client who is scheduled for surgery has already been to see a specialist to determine that the surgery is required. The surgeon's HOP will know the surgeon's schedule and will book the procedure with the appropriate facility. The surgeon's office may notify the client of the date or may notify the family doctor's office. Make sure you pass on this information to the client. Some basic information is needed in booking surgery:

- The client's name
- Address
- Phone number
- Date of birth
- Provincial/territorial health plan number
- Private insurance coverage, if any
- Type of accommodation requested if an overnight stay is required (standard/ward, semi-private, private room)
- Referring physician's name
- Surgeon's name

The client's **provisional diagnosis** will also be required, that is, the diagnosis made before the procedure is done. This diagnosis may change after the procedure. For example, a client may have a provisional diagnosis of an ovarian cyst and be booked for a laparoscopy. The procedure may reveal that she has an ectopic pregnancy.

You may need to book an appointment for a client to come in to the family physician's office for a pre-operative assessment. Clients having a major operation must have a complete assessment to provide current information about their medical

PROVISIONAL DIAGNOSIS
a tentative diagnosis made before a procedure is done, which may be confirmed or changed by findings.

conditions and to determine if they can tolerate the surgery. Most hospitals have a pre-op teaching program, usually outpatient, for surgical clients. The client will have a hospital orientation, fill out some preliminary forms, and be told what to expect before and after the operation.

Summary

1. Scheduling appointments is one of the HOP's main responsibilities and takes knowledge, judgment, and people skills.

2. Appointment books are available in various formats and should be chosen to match the needs of the practice. Computerized scheduling allows direct links with billing and is more flexible. You will often print out a copy of the day's schedule for yourself and the physician. Most practices use a printed day sheet. Make sure to note any changes or cancellations.

3. Pre-edit the appointment schedule to block off the physician's prior commitments and time off.

4. Keep appointment books confidential. If you make changes, rule a line through an entry rather than erasing it.

5. Walk-in and urgent care clinics usually have open scheduling within fixed hours. Specialists may prefer affinity booking—grouping appointments for similar purposes—and family doctors may blend affinity with random scheduling. Double booking is used to cope with a busy day and assumes that some clients will take less of the doctor's time. Stream scheduling, in which each client is assigned a specific, unique time slot, is the most common. Each method has advantages and disadvantages. You may be able to modify your office's scheduling method to enhance efficiency.

6. The time required for an appointment depends on the type of practice, the provider's style, and the reason for the visit. Typically, a minor assessment may take five to seven minutes, an intermediate assessment, 10 to 15 minutes, and a complete assessment or annual health exam, 20 to 40 minutes or longer. You need to ask the reason for the visit to book appropriately.

7. Triage is an important skill. Let someone with an urgent problem see the doctor out of turn. On the phone, direct acute emergencies to the Emergency Department. If in any doubt, consult the doctor or nurse.

8. If a client's concern is not urgent, stick to your scheduling policy. Be firm but tactful, and offer alternatives. Unless concerns are urgent, do not allow clients to bring extra family members to be seen or to discuss additional problems.

9. Scheduling catch-up time helps you deal with unpredictable events. If the physician is called away, try to contact clients to cancel appointments. Apologize and reschedule.

10. Ask new clients to come in early to fill out a health questionnaire. Consider creating a sheet or booklet outlining office hours and policies.

11. In booking specialist appointments and diagnostic tests, first find out when the client is available. Make sure the specialist gets all necessary information and that the client knows the date, location, and what to bring. In booking surgery, you may need to schedule a pre-op assessment.

Key Terms

AFFINITY (CLUSTER, CATEGORIZATION, OR ANALOGOUS) SCHEDULING 242 COMBINATION SCHEDULING OR BLENDED SCHEDULING 243	DOUBLE (DOUBLE-COLUMN) BOOKING 244 PROVISIONAL DIAGNOSIS 255	STREAM (FIXED-INTERVAL) SCHEDULING 245 WAVE SCHEDULING 242

Review Questions

1. What steps can you take to ensure that the appointment book remains confidential?

2. What is affinity scheduling, and how does it relate to stream scheduling?

3. What is meant by double booking?

4. List the advantages of using catch-up or buffer zones in the daily schedule.

5. How should you handle a client who walks into the office wanting to see the physician immediately?

6. What information should you take when booking an appointment?

7. What information should you take when booking a house call?

8. What administrative steps do you take when a new client first arrives in the office?

9. Discuss the importance of reviewing a health history with a new client.

10. What information is necessary when booking a diagnostic test such as a mammogram?

Application Exercises

1. Fill out the health history questionnaire in Figure 9.11. Review it with a peer. Were there any areas of the questionnaire that you did not complete in enough detail? Did you note allergies? If you are uncomfortable with revealing your own medical history, answer in the role of a fictitious client.

2. (a) Design an appointment book page on your computer, or choose a design from a local stationery store, suitable for the office of a primary care physician.

   (b) Pre-edit the next week, using the following information:

   i. Dr. Schumacher does hospital rounds from 8:30 a.m. to 9:30 a.m. every day.

   ii. He likes to do physical examinations in the morning on Tuesdays and Thursdays, but no more than two per day.

   iii. On Thursday, he has a client care conference 11:00–11:45 a.m. in his office.

   iv. He must be out of the office by 5:00 p.m. on Thursday for another meeting.

   v. He is seeing a drug rep 10:00–10:15 a.m. on Friday.

   (c) Book the following appointments. Assume that Dr. Schumacher's style is to take an average length of time with patients or just a little longer. For each client, consider

   ◆ what level of assessment is needed (minor, intermediate, major),

   ◆ how long an appointment to book, and

   ◆ the best time to book it.

   i. Mr. Reynolds wants to have his annual physical examination. Ph: 432-4444; e-mail: reynolds@sunshine.on.ca. Retired. At home most of the time.

   ii. Donna Kim needs an appointment for her first prenatal visit. W: 332-3432 H: 343-3333. She works full days and has three other children.

   iii. Elaine Yang is due for her allergy shot. She does not have to see Dr. Schumacher. She is at school full time. H: 332-3332.

   iv. Maya Appleton has had a cold and sore throat for three days. She has experienced a pain in her left ear for the last 24 hours. She is 13 years old. H: 222-2222.

   v. Jessica Zehr has a rash on her left forearm. Homemaker. H: 333-2222.

   vi. Mihail Reznikoff complains of diarrhea and abdominal cramps that he has had for 24 hrs. H: 333-3333 W: 333-2222.

   vii. Elisabeth Walker, who is a diabetic, has been having trouble with regulation of her blood sugar level. She states she has been hypoglycemic twice in the past three days. She also has a sore on her left foot.

   viii. Rachel Desmond is planning to become pregnant. She is coming in for advice and genetic counselling. She prefers Thursday.

   ix. Marnie McLaughlin needs an appointment for a well-baby exam for Karen, who is 3 months old. H: 222-5555. Marnie is on maternity leave. Wednesdays work best, she says.

x.   Emily Lawton is coming in for a physical examination. She is 88 years old. PH 111-2222.

xi.   Mr. Anatoly wants an appointment. His left knee is swollen, and he is having difficulty walking. H: 234-3333 W: 943-9969. Thursdays are good.

xii.   Mrs. Hazel calls and wants an immediate renewal for her Valium. H: 323-4444 W: 321-0222.

xiii.   Cathy Evans needs an appointment to discuss placing her aged mother in a nursing home. Any day is good.

xiv.   Jeremy Karsch wants an appointment for what he thinks is a recurrence of his bronchitis. e-mail: jhewitt.@sympatico.ca.

xv.   Mario Liotta wants to see the doctor. He is complaining of redness and swelling in his left leg. H. 432-3233.

xvi.   Phil Ioannou needs an allergy shot. (PH 111-2441)

xvii.   Georgina Gould wants an appointment for a gynecological examination, Pap smear, and insertion of an intrauterine contraceptive device (IUD, or IUCD). Any day but Mon./Tues. works for her. PH 426-9214.

xviii.   Gary Janacek was asked to come in today for a blood pressure check. PH 421-6666.

xix.   Betty Nguyen calls with vague symptoms of fatigue. PH 944-2111. Wants Tues. appt.

xx.   Shaundra Ladouceur comes in complaining of a plantar wart (a wart on the sole of the foot). PH 111-942. Any day is OK.

(d) In groups of three to four, compare your appointment books. Do your partners see any problems with your scheduling? In particular, note any differences in how long an appointment each of you assigned to a given client. Was this because you came to different conclusions about what level of assessment was needed? Decide as a group which level is accurate. Adjust your schedule to solve any problems pointed out by your partners.

features, including a two-character version code for replacement cards. Under the heading "Card Valid/Carte valide," the card issue and expiry dates are listed. The cardholder's birth date and gender are also given.

The Ontario photo health card was introduced in February 1995. The main reason for this was to add security features and reduce fraudulent use of the health-care system. The information on the front of the card includes the health number and version code, a digitalized signature, and the date of birth (YMD order). The version code is designed to prevent stolen or lost cards from being used fraudulently. A replacement card will have a different version code than the original. The back contains a statement on the cardholder's responsibility, a magnetic strip that allows you to check client information with a swipe, an organ donor code, a bar code for checking validity, and a holographic overlay, which is another feature to prevent counterfeiting. The photo card must be renewed when it expires. (Most health cards across Canada have expiry dates; periods range from three to five years.) Progress has been slow in replacing all cards. Residents are sent a letter notifying them that they must come in and get a photo ID card issued to them. Children under 15½ years do not have photos taken and do not need to come in. Other provinces that use photo cards also do not use photos for children before the mid-teens because their appearances change too rapidly.

Privacy and the Health Card

A health card is an important personal document that must be treated as private and confidential. It is to be used for health-care purposes only. It is illegal to ask someone to show a health card for identification purposes (e.g., cashing a cheque, applying for a charge card, proof of age). An exception is that seniors in Ontario may use their Health 65 card as proof of age for seniors' discounts. Showing the card, however, is voluntary. This does not hold true in all provinces.

Registering for Provincial/Territorial Health Insurance Coverage

You will likely be asked about registering for health coverage. Although the information is publicly available, it is helpful to understand the process so that you can explain it to clients.

Each province or territory has its own application form, usually available at doctors' offices, hospitals, and ministry offices in cities and larger towns (see your local phone book). Figure 10.2 shows an application form for Prince Edward Island. In some provinces, the form may be mailed, faxed, or brought in to the approved location along with the appropriate identification and citizenship or immigration documents.

Each applicant must supply the ministry with specific information and validate this information. This information is stored in a central electronic database and is confidential. The insured person must supply accurate, current information.

Stress the importance of bringing all the required documentation. Without it, applications will not be processed, which will lead to delays and frustration. Keep Table 10.3 handy for reference. This table shows documentation required for Ontario; similar documents are accepted in other jurisdictions. Clients are often surprised at what is accepted as documentation. Applicants need documentation from three categories, a fact that confuses many people.

Prince Edward Island

CANADA

Health & Social Services

35 Douses Road, PO Box 3000
Montague, PEI C0A 1R0
Telephone: 838-0900 or 1-800-321-5492

REGISTRATION APPLICATION

FOR OFFICE USE ONLY

DOCUMENT # _____		HOUSEHOLD # _____	
DATE ELIGIBLE	D | M | Y	STATUS _____	
DATE ENTERED	D | M | Y	ENTERED BY _____	
DATE APPROVED	D | M | Y	APPROVED BY _____	

	Birth Date (D M Y)	Sex (M/F)	Country and Province of Birth	FOR OFFICE USE ONLY
Name (surname, first name, initials)				Personal Health Number
Mailing Address	City/Town		Postal Code	
(Home) (Work) Telephone No.				
Spouse (surname, first name, initials)	Birth Date (D M Y)	Sex (M/F)	Country and Province of Birth	Personal Health Number
Dependants (surname, first name, initials) 1.	Birth Date (D M Y)	Sex (M/F)	Country and Province of Birth	Personal Health Number
2.				
3.				
4.				

List additional dependants on back of application.

Residential Status

☐ New Resident   ☐ Returning Resident   ☐ R.C.M.P., Armed Forces, Penitentiary
(Please indicate release date if any of the above apply.)   D \| M \| Y

Province/Country of last residence

Mailing Address   City/Town   Postal Code

Former Provincial Health Care No. (if applicable)

Reason for coming to Prince Edward Island

☐ Internship   ☐ Student   ☐ Employment   ☐ Other _____
(Please specify)

Length of stay on Prince Edward Island   Permanent _____   Temporary _____

Date of arrival on Prince Edward Island   D \| M \| Y

Figure 10.2 Application for health coverage in Prince Edward Island.

Table 10.3 | Documents Required to Apply for Health Insurance (Ontario)

Applicants must bring *one* document from *each of the three* following categories:

1. Proof of Canadian citizenship or immigration status
   - Birth certificate from a Canadian province, territory, or the Department of National Defence
   - Certificate of Canadian citizenship
   - Certificate of naturalization
   - Current Canadian passport
   - Certified statement of live birth from a Canadian province or territory
   - Certificate of baptism, if born in Quebec or Newfoundland prior to January 1994
   - Certificate of First Nations status
   - Immigrant visa and record of landing
   - Canadian immigration identification card
   - Canadian certificate of registration of birth abroad
   - Employment authorization

2. Proof of residency in the province or territory (varies somewhat; check the local form)
   - Valid driver's licence or temporary driver's licence
   - Ontario motor vehicle permit
   - Bank account statement (savings or chequing account, not automatic teller receipts)
   - Utility bill (telephone, cable TV, public utilities commission, hydro, gas, or water)
   - Mortgage, rental, or lease agreement
   - Income tax assessment
   - Insurance policy (home, tenant, auto, or life)
   - Employee record (pay stub)
   - Age of Majority card
   - Statement of old age security

- Statement of unemployment insurance benefits paid (T4U)
- Child tax benefit statement
- Statement of workers' compensation benefits
- Letter from First Nations band administrator
- Canada Pension Plan statement of contributions
- Statement of RRSP
- Property tax bill
- Letter from an administrator of a publicly funded, long-term care facility or an agency for Convention refugees or the homeless

3. Proof of *personal* identity (i.e., that you are who you say you are)
   - Social Insurance Number (SIN) card
   - Credit card
   - Bank card
   - Current employee ID
   - Student ID
   - Union card
   - Library card
   - Certified Statement of Marriage from the Registrar General
   - Marriage certificate
   - Valid driver's licence or temporary licence
   - Provincial motor vehicle permit
   - Certificate of Canadian citizenship
   - Passport (Canadian or foreign)
   - Canadian immigration identification card
   - Current professional association licence
   - Certificate of First Nations status
   - Old Age Security card
   - Ontario Ministry of Natural Resources Outdoors card

Note that some documents appear in more than one category. However, you cannot use the same document twice in the registration process (e.g., if you use your driver's licence for one section, you cannot use it again for another section). The Ministry will not accept affidavits and statutory declarations or waive a document requirement. You may be asked for additional documentation (e.g., if your name has changed).

Temporary Health Cards

In most provinces, a paper health card similar to the plastic card is issued for clients who need a card immediately (for example, those whose cards are lost or stolen) or who are eligible for coverage for only a short period of time. In some provinces, a validated copy of the application form accepted by the ministry serves as a temporary card.

Registering Newborns

When a baby is born, the birth must be registered. Newborn registration must be completed before a birth certificate can be issued. Newborns are covered immediately by provincial/territorial health insurance plans in the province of residence provided (in most provinces) that at least one parent is eligible to receive health care in that province. In some jurisdictions, including Ontario, hospitals and midwives have forms with pre-assigned health numbers, which they complete when a baby is born. There is

GOVERNMENT OF NEWFOUNDLAND AND LABRADOR
Department of Health and Community Services

mcp

NEWBORN / ADOPTED CHILD REGISTRATION FORM
Please Print

MAILING ADDRESS

Street/P.O. Box	City/Town	
Province	Postal Code	Telephone Number (Home)	Telephone Number (Work)

PARENT OR GUARDIAN

MCP Registration Number	Surname	Given Name and Initials	Birth Date (YY/MM/DD)

CHILD/CHILDREN TO BE REGISTERED

Surname	Given Name and Initials	Sex (M/F)	Birth Date (YY/MM/DD)

DECLARATION (It is an offense to give false information for the purpose of obtaining coverage under the Newfoundland and Labrador Medical Care Plan)

I hereby declare that the information given is correct and the person(s) listed on this form are residents of Newfoundland and Labrador.

Signature   Date

REQUIRED DOCUMENTATION

If registering a child/children through adoption, a copy of the official adoption papers, or the birth certificate, is required for each child.

If the surname of the child/children is different than the registering parent or guardian, a copy of the birth certificate is required for each child.

Medical Care Plan
22 High Street, P. O. Box 5000
Grand Falls-Windsor NL Canada A2A 2Y4
Tel: 1-800-563-1557 Fax: 709-292-4052

http://www.gov.nf.ca/mcp

Medical Care Plan
57 Margaret's Place, P. O. Box 8700
St. John's NL Canada A1B 4J6
Tel: 1-800-563-1557 Fax: 709-758-1694

Figure 10.3 Application to register a newborn or adopted child in Newfoundland and Labrador.

CHAPTER 11

Preparing for the Billing Process

LEARNING OBJECTIVES

On completing this chapter, you will be able to:

1. Explain how ministries monitor the validity of submitted claims.

2. Discuss three methods of health card validation.

3. State the benefits of health card validation.

4. Respond appropriately to clients who do not have valid health cards.

5. Explain the function of physician registration numbers and the structure of Ontario numbers.

6. Explain the structure of Ontario service codes.

7. Distinguish among general, intermediate, and minor assessments.

8. Recognize the purpose and usefulness of the ICD system.

9. Explain when to use premium codes.

Chapter 10 gave an overview of health coverage, especially provincial/territorial coverage. This chapter explains the principles of billing. General rules and policies are similar across Canada, as are definitions for such things as an encounter, consultation, and a comprehensive visit. All provinces and territories use physician numbers, service codes, and diagnostic codes, discussed in this chapter. Chapter 12 will describe specific billing procedures using current software.

The Claims Review Process

A health claim is submitted to a provincial/territorial plan in much the same way as you would submit a claim to any insurance company. The body or bodies responsible for health insurance are the payment agencies. They accept, approve, monitor, and sometimes investigate claims and participate in deciding what services are insured.

The cycle of provincial/territorial billing for the HOP *begins* with the submission of a claim for services rendered. The ministry then reviews the claim, and the cycle ends with payment to the provider for all valid claims. The ministry examines each claim submitted to ensure that

◆ the provider has a valid billing number,

◆ the service claimed is authorized by provincial/territorial guidelines,

◆ the fee claimed is the one determined by the fee schedule,

◆ the client has a valid health card, and

◆ the claim is submitted in a technically correct manner.

All claims must be submitted in a certain format and within a designated time frame.

Claims Monitoring and Control

All provinces and territories use similar methods to monitor fee-for-service claims submitted. The monitoring body (usually the Ministry of Health) must ensure that claims are made properly and that payments are for health services authorized by provincial/territorial guidelines. The monitoring process helps identify irregularities and fraud.

Inappropriate billing by organizations and physicians and the fraudulent use of health cards are ongoing problems that cost the provincial/territorial plans dearly. All claims submitted are routinely subjected to computer checks, and if they do not meet health plan requirements, they may be rejected or only partially paid. Selected claims may be forwarded to a medical review committee to determine whether the claim is valid and should be paid. Periodically, physicians will be asked for copies of their records.

Ministries investigate reports of inappropriate billing promptly and thoroughly. Both the medical associations and the ministries may take disciplinary action.

Ministries also try to reduce invalid claims by educating and supporting physicians and their administrative staff. Most jurisdictions have a regional information service to answer questions and provide clarification. Contact this service if you are not sure whether a service is insured or how to submit a particular claim.

Each province/territory also has a list of health services that must be reviewed individually and approved in advance. Breast reduction is one example. If the proposal is rejected and the client still wants the service, she must pay for it. A physician who fails to seek approval for a service in this category risks not being paid for it. Clients also need prior approval to seek some treatments outside their own province or territory.

Verification Letters

Some jurisdictions have a verification letter program to audit providers' billing activities. Computer-generated letters are sent randomly to clients, who are asked to verify that the physician actually provided the service he billed for. (Letters will not be sent about services that clients may regard as especially private, such as abortion; treatment of sexually transmitted diseases, AIDS, or dementia; assessment of genitalia; or organ retrieval after death.) Individually prepared letters may also be sent to the clients of physicians who are under review or are suspected of inappropriate or fraudulent billing. Verification letters are intended primarily to uncover fraud, to monitor claims under investigation, and to document fraud already identified. In addition, they make the public aware of the costs of health services. Under special circumstances, a physician can request that a client not receive such a letter if she believes it would not be in the client's best interests.

Example: On January 3, Jim Dobryn went to the doctor complaining of abdominal pain. The physician completed a full assessment based on the initial findings. A month later, Jim received a letter from the ministry stating that the physician had been reimbursed for a check-up on January 3 and asking Jim to let the Ministry of Health know, in writing or by telephone, whether this check-up took place. If Jim had called to say he never had such a check-up, the doctor would have been investigated.

Implications for the HOP

A client may call your office with questions regarding such a letter. If the client is confused about the letter, clarify its purpose. If he is not sure how to respond, tell him that the letter should contain a phone number and address. Do not question the client about the specific content of the letter. Often, the client will remember coming to the office but not remember the date or time. Confirm this information by looking in the client's chart.

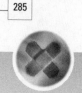

Health Card Validation

Some provinces try to control health card fraud by using health cards that have expiry dates and that incorporate photographs and version codes. As emphasized in Chapter 10, clients should always present a health card before receiving a medical service. Health card validation (HCV) means checking the card to make sure that it is authentic, current, and matches your information for the client. This confirms that the client is eligible to receive the service.

You may feel that validating every card is a waste of your time and the client's time. However, the process offers real benefits for both the provider and the health system. The health-care system benefits because validation reduces the fraudulent use of cards. You benefit because you significantly reduce rejected claims. (Invalid cards are one of the most common reasons for claims rejection). This improves your provider's cash flow and saves the time and expense of sorting out and resubmitting rejected claims. You are also prompted to verify the client's current address, which keeps your records up-to-date. Although you should validate all cards, the process is especially important for out-of-town clients, new clients, and referred clients you do not know personally.

Note: Any HCV system needs to be secure because it grants query access to the Registered Persons Database, which contains confidential information such as health card numbers. Most ministries require that users have a password, which must be changed periodically. In Ontario, a password is valid for 38 days. *Keep track of when your password expires, and change it before it does.* Keep it confidential; if you write it down, ensure that only you have access to it.

> **INSIST THAT CLIENTS PRESENT THEIR HEALTH CARD *BEFORE* A SERVICE IS RENDERED. VALIDATE THE HEALTH CARD AT EACH VISIT.**

Methods of Validation

There are several ways that you can validate a client's health card. Which will suit you best depends on the size of your practice or clinic, the speed of response required, and whether your clients are mostly long term or transient and booked in advance or walk-in. Efficient validation methods are part of most primary care reform initiatives. The following is a summary of the more commonly used validation systems.

Overnight Batch Eligibility Checking (OBEC)

This method, available to those who submit claims electronically, uses **electronic data transfer** to validate health cards the day before the client is seen. You submit an electronic file to the ministry containing each client's name, health card number, and version code. This file is checked overnight and deposited in your "pick-up box" for review the next morning. This process takes little of your time, making it particularly attractive if you have a high client volume. Although effective, it only validates clients who have made appointments for a service ahead of time. Therefore, it would not work well in a walk-in clinic or an office that takes a lot of same-day bookings. When the ministry is busy with end-of-month processing, the validation may take longer than overnight.

ELECTRONIC DATA TRANSFER exchanging information electronically between computers in a process similar to e-mail; a common method of claims submission.

Interactive Voice Response

Interactive voice response (IVR) is a popular choice for smaller practices. This is an automated method of health card validation that is available 24 hours a day, seven days a week, using a touch-tone phone to call a toll-free number.

◆ Key in your personal identification number (PIN). This ensures that the information exchanged remains confidential.

- ◆ You will then be asked to key in the health card number and the version code of the card you are validating.
- ◆ A pre-recorded, coded response will notify you whether the card is valid.
- ◆ You can also access bulletins posted by the ministry.

This system is inexpensive and does not have to be integrated into the office's software system. Another advantage is that it allows you to enter a fee schedule code to determine whether a client is eligible for a service, such as a routine check-up or a visual examination, that is covered only once in a given period. For example, suppose your province allows check-ups every two years. Sally has booked a routine check-up on September 12, but her two years will not be up until January 18. You will be given this date, and can offer Sally the option of rescheduling or, under certain circumstances, of paying for the service herself if she does not want to wait. However, IVR does tie up the telephone line and takes up your time since the process is manual.

Health Card Reader (HCR)/Point-of-Service Device

A range of devices, called magnetic card readers or point of service (POS) devices, are available for health card validation. Some stand alone; others are integrated into the office's software.

STAND-ALONE DEVICES The stand-alone POS device uses a dedicated phone line and is much like the one stores and restaurants use for processing credit card purchases. You swipe the health card and the device reads the information on the card's magnetic strip and transmits it to the ministry's computer. The validity of the health card is assessed and a response sent back.

PC POS DEVICE The PC point of service device uses a standard PC with a modem and special software. A card is swiped in a wedge device (Figure 11.1) that attaches to the computer keyboard. If the health card is not available, the number can be entered using the keyboard. This process can be integrated within a client registration system or run in a Windows environment in conjunction with other applications. The software enables the PC to submit the card data and receive a response from the ministry's health card validation service. A patient's health card status is also updated as billings are accepted using the stored health card information. This ensures that a patient's health card status is always as up-to-date as possible. Figure 11.2 shows a return message noting a valid card and client information.

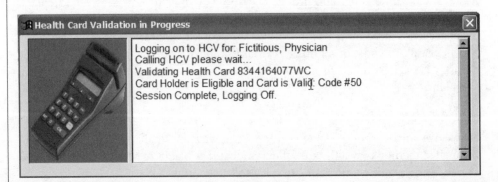

Figure 11.1   Magnetic card reader and response.

Visual Practice Software image supplied courtesy of Advanced Computer Systems Limited.

♦ an examination of one or more body parts (the affected body part(s), system(s), or mental or emotional disorder, as needed to establish a diagnosis) or direct further tests to establish a diagnosis.

In B.C., a similar service is called a partial/regional examination.

Consider two other examples of intermediate assessments:

Arlene comes into Dr. Tran's office complaining of vague gastrointestinal, symptoms including diarrhea and epigastric burning (a burning sensation below the sternum, or breastbone). Dr. Tran does a related history about her eating and bowel habits. He asks some questions related to the cardiovascular system. He does an abdominal examination, perhaps a rectal examination as well, and listens to the heart and chest. This would constitute an intermediate assessment because the doctor took a detailed history of the complaint, made inquiries regarding the cardiovascular system and the respiratory system, and examined the gastrointestinal, cardiovascular, and respiratory systems.

Paul arrives complaining of an earache and a sore throat. Dr. Lyons examines his ears, throat, and lymph nodes, and probably listens to his chest and takes vital signs. She takes a related history. This would also be an intermediate assessment because the doctor examined more than one system (ears, throat, lymph glands, and the respiratory system) and asked questions related to each system.

Well Baby

(Code A007 Dx 916)

A *well-baby visit* is considered an intermediate assessment. This involves routine periodic assessment during the first two years of life. It includes a complete examination, with weight and measurements, and instructions to the parent(s) or caregiver regarding related health care and health teaching and appropriate immunizations covered routinely by OHIP. The same code is used whether a parent brings a child under two years into the office for a routine check-up or because of a physical complaint, but a diagnostic code of 916 is used for a well-baby visit.

Annual Health/Physical Examination (Child)

(Code K017—no diagnostic code needed)

This is a general assessment of a child two to 15 years of age who does not present with health problems. It includes all relevant instructions and health teaching. This assessment code includes primary and secondary school examinations.

Minor Assessment

(Code A001)

A minor assessment is also considered a primary care assessment and is used frequently in the doctor's office. This code is used when the encounter involves a brief history, examination of the affected part or region or mental or emotional disorder, and/or brief advice or information regarding health maintenance, diagnosis, treatment, or prognosis.

Examples of a minor assessment:

Trudy had been diagnosed with pneumonia and was treated with an antibiotic for 10 days. She comes back in so that Dr. Dumont can quickly assess her recovery. He asks her how she is feeling, if she has any shortness of breath, fever, and so on. He listens to her chest and, finding nothing, concludes the assessment.

Victor is going abroad and comes in to see Dr. Dumont to ask what immunizations he will need.

Mei-Lin has been having trouble with a skin rash, and Dr. Dumont prescribed some new medication for it. She comes in so that he can assess her progress. He checks her rash, asks a couple of questions, and concludes the assessment.

Mini Assessment

(Code A008)

This code is used if the docor has to examine the client for a completely unrelated problem during the same office visit for an examination of a WSIB assessment. An A008 can only be claimed in conjunction with a WSIB claim for which the WSIB will only pay for a minor assessment during the same visit.

General Assessment for a Prenatal Visit

(Code P003)

This is usually the initial assessment once an initial diagnosis of pregnancy has been established. This visit is more detailed than subsequent visits and requires a detailed history and physical assessment of the mother-to-be and related health teaching.

Prenatal Office Visits

(Code P004)

This code is used for subsequent prenatal visits after the initial more complete prenatal assessment. These visits are for a routine pregnancy are specific and do not involve an in-depth assessment. The assessment primarily includes testing a urine sample for protein, glucose, and acetone, taking the woman's weight and vital signs, taking fetal heart rate (once audible), measuring the height of the **fundus**, asking a range of related questions, and answering any concerns the woman might have.

FUNDUS the top of the uterus. Measuring how high the fundus is in the abdomen provides valuable information about the size of the uterus and the progression of fetal growth.

ANTENATAL before birth.

Antenatal Preventative Health Assessment

(Code P005)

This new code is used for a client who is considering pregnancy. The physician conducts an examination, reviews the client's history, and assesses genetic, psychosocial, and medical risks. This assessment may be conducted once per pregnancy and may not be conducted on the same day as a general prenatal assessment (P003) or prenatal office visit (P004). The documentation must be part of the client's permanent record.

Attendance at Labour and Delivery

(Code P009)

This new code may be used for assisting with a vaginal delivery or cesarean section, giving anesthetic for a Caesarean section or **operative delivery** (e.g., use of forceps), or for newborn resuscitation. This service will have a premium added.

OPERATIVE DELIVERY the delivery of a baby that involves the use of any assistive devices, such as forceps; in contrast to a *spontaneous delivery*, in which the mother pushes the baby out without assistance.

Newborn Care

(Code H001)

This code, for routine care of a baby up to 10 days of age, includes initial general assessment and subsequent assessments, including instructions to the parent(s) regarding basic health care. The service usually involves two visits but may involve only one for those clients whose hospital stay is less than 24 hours. Only one doctor may claim newborn care for a given baby. For example, if a pediatrician renders care, the family doctor may not claim the same service. A family doctor may, however, claim for newborn care for a baby delivered by an obstetrician. Midwives will provide newborn care for the babies they deliver if the babies are healthy.

Individual Counselling

(Code K013)

This is defined as a visit to discuss the client's problems and help the client develop an awareness of them and consider solutions. If this discussion involves two or more individuals, it is classified as *group counselling* and is coded as K040 or K041. Remuneration for counselling is based on time units. One unit of time is equal to half an hour. If a counselling session lasts less than 20 minutes, the session should be claimed as an intermediate or minor assessment, whichever is most appropriate. If the counselling session lasts more than a half hour, extra time is calculated and claimed using the code K033.

In B.C., the criteria for counselling services by a family doctor are somewhat stricter. The problem must be considered by the physician to be "medically difficult," must cause the client "significant" distress, and must require extended advice or discussion. In most provinces, clients with more serious emotional/mental problems and psychiatric diseases are referred to specialists.

Services to Hospital Inpatients

In all provinces, physicians attend to clients within the hospital setting. Increasingly, particularly in larger settings, this is done by consultants. Family physicians in some jurisdictions also carry out minor procedures in the hospital and may treat clients in the emergency room. Each province will have service codes for services provided to clients in hospital, both inpatients and outpatients. If you are working for a general practitioner, it is your responsibility to ensure that all claims for hospital visits and procedures are submitted.

The prefix C is used for all nonemergency services to inpatients in acute care hospitals. All claims for visits to clients in hospital must show an admission date. The service code for an initial visit and in-hospital assessment (normally on the admission date) is C003. Any subsequent visit—a routine assessment on another day— is coded C002. A maximum of one visit per day per client is allowed.

Special Service Code Notifiers

UVC stands for Use Visit Code. Beside some items in the Schedule of Benefits is the code UVC instead of a specific procedural code. Do not claim for these items separately; they are considered to be part of a visit. For example, removing a Shirodkar suture (a stitch put into a woman's cervix to prevent spontaneous abortion) is marked UVC in the schedule. You would not submit a claim for this procedure but would simply bill the appropriate code for the office visit during which the stitch was removed.

IC stands for Independent Consideration. Independent consideration may be given when a set fee is not listed in the Schedule of Benefits. The District Marshall Consultant reviews each such claim individually. These claims must be sent with a letter and either an operative report or a consultation report detailing relevant data.

Diagnostic and Therapeutic Procedural Codes

This grouping refers to diagnostic procedures, such as ultrasounds, pulmonary function tests, biopsies, aspirations, scopes, and so on (see Table 11.4). Injections and urine testing in the office would also be included in this category. They are represented by the prefix G. The physician may claim with the appropriate service code as well as the related procedure code *unless the procedure is the only reason for the visit*. If the procedure is the only reason for the visit, the listed value for the procedure will apply. For example, if a client comes in for an allergy shot and nothing else, then only the procedural code is applied. If a client comes in complaining of an earache and also has an allergy shot at the same visit, then the doctor can claim for the office visit and assessment related to the earache and for the allergy shot.

Sometimes, a diagnostic code is necessary, and sometimes it is not. Some software systems will not accept a procedural code without a diagnostic code. Some procedures, such as a flu vaccine and other immunizations, have specific diagnostic codes that are used with them. Others, such as a urinalysis, if done in the office, do not usually require a diagnostic code. If the software system must have a diagnostic code, use the diagnostic code that reflects the condition or suspected condition for which the test is being done.

The Diagnostic Code

The diagnostic code represents the physician's diagnosis of the client's condition on which treatment decisions are based. In examining the client, the doctor looks for clinical signs or symptoms that suggest a diagnosis. Some sets of symptoms are specific and point clearly to a particular diagnosis; others are more ambiguous and more open to interpretation. If the doctor cannot clearly pinpoint a diagnosis, she can choose general descriptive terms such as "Respiratory symptoms not yet diagnosed (NYD)," or even, when nothing really fits, "Other ill-defined conditions."

Most claims require that the diagnosis be identified. This may be done using a specified code format or by submitting the actual diagnosis on the claim form. For those health plans using a diagnostic code, this ensures that the service the provider has claimed is appropriate for the client's diagnosis. Diagnostic codes are virtually the same across Canada; they are based on the International Classification of Diseases (ICD) coding system. Many provinces have now adopted the most recent version, ICD 10, or are in the process of converting to this system. The code usually consists of three numeric characters. Table 11.4 lists common diagnostic codes. In Figure 11.3, the diagnostic code is 460. Table 11.5 lists definitions of common terms used in relation to diagnoses and services.

Certain diagnostic codes will normally accompany certain service codes. For example, diagnostic code 388 (wax in the ears) goes with procedural code G420 (syringing the ear). Diagnostic code 477 (hay fever, rhinitis) often accompanies allergy injections (G202 or G212). Diagnostic code 487 accompanies flu vaccine (G590 or G591). The Ministry of Health uses the 487 code to track the number of flu shots given.

A few service codes (e.g., K107) do not require diagnostic codes. Some procedures require a diagnostic code; others do not. However, some billing software (discussed in Chapter 12) will not accept a procedural code without a diagnostic code. In this case, use the diagnostic code for the condition or suspected condition for which the test is being done.

A pronouncement of death includes a diagnostic code, which should be the code for the cause of death listed on the death certificate. This should be the underlying, rather than the immediate, cause of death. For example, if a client suffering from chronic obstructive pulmonary disease (COPD) died of heart failure caused by the lung disease, the diagnostic code would be 496 for COPD, the underlying cause.

Time Units

Time units are most often used for specialists such as surgeons and anesthetists. Most, but not all, codes with the B suffix are billed in units of time. For example, 15 minutes might be one time unit. An hour would be four time units. Sometimes, a hardship benefit may apply after a certain point. For example, suppose the time unit is 15 minutes and the cut-off point is two hours; the hardship point allows doubling the units. For example, a doctor assisting with a surgical procedure is allowed three hours. The total number of units should actually be 12 (3 hours × 4 time units). However, you would count the first two hours as eight units, and then double the units in the last hour to count as another eight units, producing a total of 16. In most provinces, there is also a

Key Terms

ANTENATAL 300	ELECTRONIC DATA TRANSFER 285	PHYSICIAN REGISTRATION
BILLING (SERVICE, ITEM) CODE 290	FUNDUS 300	NUMBER 288
ELECTIVE SURGERY 298	OPERATIVE DELIVERY 300	SPECIALIST 289
	OXYTOCIN DRIP 309	

Review Questions

1. How do health ministries monitor claims to ensure that they are valid?

2. Compare and contrast the advantages and disadvantages of the three methods of health card validation noted in this chapter.

3. What is the purpose of the version code found on Ontario health cards?

4. What options do you have if a client has forgotten his health card?

5. What steps should you take if you suspect you have been presented with a fraudulent health card?

6. Dr. Benson's Ontario physician identification number is 4444-123459-90. Explain what each of the three components represents.

7. A007A is a service code. Explain the code, considering the prefix, numeric component, and suffix.

8. Identify a situation where you would use a diagnostic code with a procedural code.

9. Explain claims marked IC and those marked UVC in the Schedule of Benefits.

10. What is a premium code? In general terms, when would you use premium codes?

Application Exercises

1. Independently, or with a peer, think of effective ways to encourage clients to present their health cards. Consider a creative sign for the reception area. Plan two responses to clients who repeatedly do not update their health card information or who leave their cards at home.

2. Marty is 70 years old and lives in Spruce Lodge, a nursing home. The nurses call Dr. Thompson at 0200 to say that Marty is short of breath and complaining of feeling weak. Dr. Thompson arrives at 0230.

   a. What service code would you use?

   b. What premium code would you use?

3. For each of the following scenarios, fill in the service code, procedural code (if applicable), diagnostic code (if applicable), and premium code (if applicable). Use the sites listed under Web Sites of Interest and/or the tables in this chapter.

   a. Leigh came in to see the doctor complaining of an earache in the left ear. She was also having difficulty swallowing. The doctor examined her ears, looked at her throat, and listened to her chest. He took a detailed history relating to her complaint and asked questions about her respiratory system. He diagnosed otitis media and tonsillitis and sent her home with a seven-day prescription of antibiotics.

   b. Ivan came in because he was experiencing lower back pain. The doctor obtained a detailed history related to the complaint and noted on the chart that Sam also had dysuria and was febrile. A urine sample was tested in the office. The doctor diagnosed cystitis and prescribed antibiotics.

   c. Bill came to the doctor and complained of a skin rash on his forearm. The doctor looked at it and asked some questions related to the complaint. She quickly diagnosed contact dermatitis.

   d. Kersti came in complaining of a sore stomach and diarrhea. The doctor completed a history about the complaint and related system. He examined her abdomen. He concluded that she had the flu.

   e. Ardelle came in with her one-year-old son Zachary for a well-baby check-up.

   f. Ravi came for an annual medical.

g. Latoya came in for an allergy shot. The nurse gave it to her. She did not see the doctor.

h. Mrs. Purves came in for her annual physical examination. Mrs. Purves is 90 years old.

i. Gregory came in complaining of dysuria (pain on voiding), low back pain, and some hematuria (blood in the urine). The doctor diagnosed pyelonephritis and started Gregory on an anti-biotic. He also had the nurse complete a dipstick urinalysis in the office.

j. Agnes Morrow called the office and asked you to see if the doctor could come visit her after office hours. She was bedridden and had noted some increased shortness of breath. The doctor made the house call at 2000.

Item Code	PPU	Units	Type	Date	Diag. Code	MR	Amount	Status Acct#	Err.
a.									
b.									
c.									
d.									
e.									
f.									
g.									
h.									
i.									
j.									

Web Sites of Interest

Provincial Health Care in Canada
http://canadanews.about.com/cs/provhealthcare/
   index/htm

British Columbia Health Care
http://www/hlth.gov.bc.ca/msp/infoben/
   premium.htpl

BC Medical Services Commission Payment Schedule
http://www.hlth.gov.bc.ca/msp/infoprac/
   physbilling/payschedule/index.html

Alberta Health Care
http://www.health.gov.ab.ca/ahcip

Alberta Schedule of Medical Benefits
http://www.health.gov.ab.ca/professionals/
   somb.htm

Alberta Medical Association
http://www.albertadoctors.org/home/

Saskatchewan Fee Manual
http://www.health.gov.sk.ca/msb_phy_pymt_sch/
    Physician%20Payment%20Schedule%20-
    %20Updated%20March%2031%202002.pdf

Ontario Schedule of Benefits
http://www.gov.on.ca/health/english/program/
    ohip/sob/physserv/physserv_mn.html

Newfoundland and Labrador Medical Care
Plan Fees
http://www.gov.nf.ca/mcp/act_reg/regs_2.pdf

ICD-9 Diagnostic Codes
http://neuro3.stanford.edu/CodeWorrier/
http://icd9cm.chrisendres.com/index.
    php?srchtype=diseases&srchtext=
    785&action=search

These two sites allow you to enter a diagnosis and
find the code, or enter a code and find the
diagnosis.

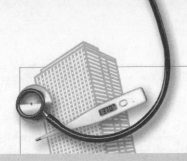

CHAPTER 12
Billing

Chapter 10 outlined the provincial and territorial health-care plans; Chapter 11 introduced the elements of billing. This chapter discusses the actual process of claims submission and the technologies available to facilitate it, as well as outlining approaches to billing payers other than provincial/territorial health plans.

The billing process is the same in all provinces and territories. The basic billing cycle is relatively simple: you collect information needed for a claim, store the claims forms on your information system, put the files together, and send them to the ministry responsible. The ministry reviews your claims according to a schedule and reports which ones are approved and which are rejected. The ministry sends payment to the provider. You have an opportunity to review, correct, and resubmit rejected claims. Throughout this chapter, Ontario examples are used. The terms used, the billing and diagnostic codes applied, the timing of claims submission/payment, and the names of the forms may be slightly different in your jurisdiction, but you will be going through the same steps in the same order. The preamble to your jurisdiction's fee schedule will give more details. It is important to know your way around the schedule and use it when in doubt. You may find it easiest to use online.

Claims Submission: The Process

The mechanics of submission is primarily the HOP's responsibility. You need to be familiar with the method of claims submission used by your provider. Even if you are familiar with the general process of claims submission, when you start a new job, you will need some orientation to the particular system. Be sure that you are comfortable

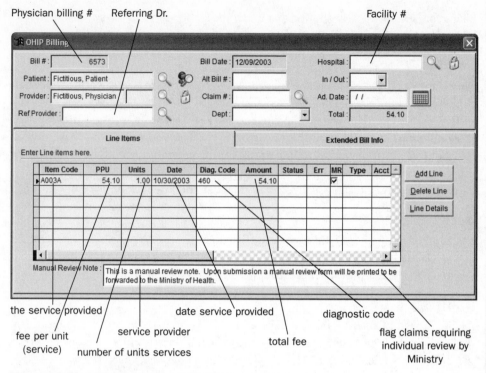

Figure 12.5 Billing screen showing coding.

Visual Practice Software image supplied courtesy of Advanced Computer Systems Limited.

surgical procedure that took longer than usual, you would need to explain the circumstances. Figure 12.5 shows a screen with a space for such an explanation. Some programs have a manual review feature that will support the entry of review comments for printing at the time of submission.

Independent Consideration

Some services are marked as IC in the Schedule of Benefits. (Some jurisdictions may use a different symbol.) This means "independent consideration," and such claims are also reviewed manually. This is sometimes referred to as being marked with a "Y" indicator. If you submit claims electronically, remember that you must fax the supporting documentation when you submit that claim. If your claims are submitted on disk or tape, send the supporting documentation the same time you send the tape or disk.

Shadow Billing

Shadow billing is used in practices that have entered into primary care reform agreements, such as family health networks. It facilitates direct comparison of the capitation fee the ministry is paying the provider with the costs that would be incurred if the provider were billing fee-for-service. Precisely how this billing is formatted may vary. There may be a special code used for rostered clients and a shadow billing option on the computer software system. For rostered clients, you will enter other information as usual but click the "shadow" tab. A zero balance is submitted. Not all software programs have this option. In some provinces, billings are done for rostered clients as if they were fee-for-service, and the ministry's computer identifies them and separates them from fee-for-service clients.

EXAMPLE Dr. Chen is working in a primary care reform group. In one calendar year, she was paid $300 000 under the capitation formula to take care of 2000 clients while providing extended hours and other health-care services to her clients. The shadow billing for her practice year showed that under the fee-for-service system, she would have billed the Ministry of Health $350 000. In this case, capitation saved the ministry $50 000.

Service Date

This is the date the service was provided. Make sure it is accurate. An incorrect date could result in the claim being rejected. Generally, it is best to process claims every day so that the service date will be the current date—which your software program will show automatically. However, there may be days when you just do not have time to complete the claims. If you are doing claims for the previous business day or if, for any other reason, you are claiming for a service provided earlier, be sure to change the service date manually. You can usually select a calendar and just click on the date you want.

Service Code

As described in Chapter 11, this is the code that identifies the type of service or encounter that is claimed and generates the amount charged for the claim. In Figure 12.5, the service code is A003A, which means an intermediate assessment in Ontario.

Diagnostic Code

As discussed in Chapter 11, this is usually a three- or four-character code that indicates the diagnosis made at the time the service was rendered. If there is more than one diagnosis, use the primary one. In Figure 12.5, the diagnostic code is 460, which refers to a cold or acute nasopharyngitis. Diagnostic codes are discussed in more detail later in the chapter.

Number of Services

The number of services refers to the number of encounters the client has had with the physician. Usually, the number of services is 1. For example, Chad visits the doctor in the office because of an earache. The doctor assesses and treats Chad. That is one service or encounter. (If Chad also mentions that his knee is troubling him, the provider cannot bill for two assessments. If the doctor performs both an intermediate and a minor assessment, bill for the intermediate assessment.) However, as noted in Chapter 11, you may claim for a number of services if they are on consecutive days for inpatients in health-care facilities. For example, if Helga was in hospital for five days, the most responsible physician (MRP) might visit her daily. You would submit a single claim for five services. However, you would submit separate claims for visits that are not on consecutive days (e.g., you would submit separate claims for a visit on November 9 and one on November 11). Some software systems require that the number of services consist of two digits. If there are fewer than 10, use a zero (thus, the most common entry is 01). For other software systems this is irrelevant. You may enter the number of services as they appear (e.g., 1.3). Provincial billing software will customize the format as required.

PPU, or Price per Unit

For most services, a "unit" is the service, and the price per unit is the amount allowed in the fee schedule for that service. For time-based services, a unit is the amount of time designated in the fee schedule; for example, a unit of time might be designated as 15 minutes. Each 15-minute period spent with a client would be worth a certain value. Extra units sometimes have a different code from that for the base unit.

In Figure 12.5, the service is A003, an intermediate assessment. The fee for this assessment is $54.10; this is the PPU.

Fee Submitted

This is the amount paid for the service provided and relates directly to the service code submitted for a particular encounter. The amounts are listed in the Schedule of

Benefits/Tariffs. In Ontario, there may be a maximum of nine digits. Your software program may automatically insert the fee when you enter the service code.

For most services, the fee submitted will be the same as the price per unit, as shown in Figure 12.5. However, if more than one service is claimed, as in consecutive hospital visits, or if the service is a time-based one and the provider spent more than one unit of time, the fee will be the price per unit times the number of services.

The input required for the health plan's computer uses neither dollar signs nor decimals. Thus, $27.05 would be simply 2705. However, as with birthdate formats, your program may show prices in a more reader-friendly format but will convert them to the required format before submitting.

Types of Claims

Physicians submit three types of claims to the provincial/territorial plan, which correspond to the payment programs discussed above. The majority of claims apply to the health-care plan itself; the others are reciprocal billing (RMB) and workers' compensation claims.

Reciprocal Claims

The reciprocal billing format is the same across Canada. If your office is computerized, you will claim for out-of-province clients just as if you were billing your own health-care plan except that you need to make sure that RMB is selected as the payment program. Also check that the client's province of origin appears in the appropriate field. Usually, the software will automatically insert the province code when you swipe the card; if it does not, insert it manually. (See Table 10.2 for a list of two-letter province codes.)

If you bill manually, use a reciprocal claims form. Double-check your form to be sure that you have included the following:

- The code of the province or territory
- The client's health card number or the equivalent
- The client's name, gender, and date of birth
- The client's home address
- Payment program (RMB)
- Payee (P)

Always validate the client's health card, as discussed in Chapter 11. If the card is not valid, charge the client, and let her know she can seek reimbursement from her home province or territory when her eligibility is re-established. Most plans will not accept reciprocal claims submitted after 90 days.

Services Excluded from RMB

Check to see that the service in question is covered under RMB. Some services, even though they may be covered by your jurisdiction, are excluded from RMB. If the client is not willing to wait to have the service done in his home province, bill the client directly. Some of the more common excluded services are as follows:

- Cosmetic surgery
- Sex reassignment surgery
- Therapeutic abortion
- Annual health exams or physicals and periodic ocular assessments

- In-vitro fertilization and artificial insemination
- Lithotripsy for gallstones
- Acupuncture, acupressure, hypnotherapy services to individuals covered by other agencies such as WSIB, Veterans' Affairs
- Genetic screening

WCB Claims (WSIB in Ontario)

Workers' compensation claims, as discussed in Chapter 10, relate to on-the-job injuries. In Ontario, and most other provinces, the Ministry of Health acts as a payment agency for the WCB or WSIB. Doctors submit workers' compensation claims directly to the local Ministry of Health, as long as the client has valid provincial health coverage. The billing is the same as for provincial claims except that you must make sure the payment program selected is WCB.

If a client cannot produce a valid health card, the provider would bill the WSIB directly. Physicians must bill the WSIB directly for services not covered by the health-care plan, such as medical–legal reports or office interviews with WSIB representatives, and for selected services noted in the Schedule of Benefits. In Ontario, providers other than physicians, such as chiropractors, chiropodists, osteopaths, optometrists, private physiotherapists, private occupational therapists, dentists, audiologists, and pharmacists, bill the WSIB directly for claims. Out-of-province physicians, opted-out physicians, and private laboratories also bill directly.

In Ontario, when a doctor assesses a client for a workers' compensation matter and also provides a service for an unrelated problem at the same visit, you submit the claim separately. Provided that the WSIB claim is for a minor assessment, the other service is claimed using the service code A008, for a mini assessment.

Sending in Claims

Claims in the health office are stored or filed on the computer. When you want to submit the claims, you *batch* them, or prepare them for submission. The process will vary with the software program. Once a batch of files has been prepared for submission, your computer will notify you that the files are ready (Figure 12.6). You then copy the files to a disk or activate the electronic file transfer process.

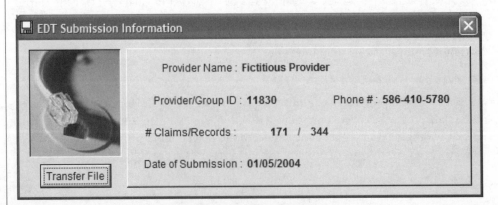

Figure 12.6   Screen indicating that batch of claims is ready to transmit.

SLI STABILITY LIFE INSURANCE COMPANY

PO Box 12345
Edmonton, AB
T3G 5N6
780-564-2929

January 26, 2004

Dear: Dr. Linh

Re: John Doe Contract 2344   **Claim 12344 – Member ID 456789**

We are writing in regards to John Doe's claim for Long Term Disability benefits.

We last received your update in November 2003 with information including consultation reports up to the end of December 2003. Please provide us with all consultation reports you have on file after December 1, 2003. In addition, in order for us to determine how his reported condition affects his ability to function and what his physical restrictions are at present, please complete the enclosed Physical Capacities Evaluation form. We have enclosed an authorization for the release of this information. Please include your correspondence fee with your reply. We would appreciate receiving a response prior to January 30, 2004.

Thank you for your assistance in this regard.

Yours truly,

JR Benesh

JR Benesh,
Disability Adjudicator,
Stability Life Insurance Company

/jb
encl

Figure 12.9   Covering letter from insurance company requesting medical records and form completion.

Table 12.2 summarizes the process of billing health-care plans.

Table 12.2 | Summary of Health-Care Plan Billing

Methods

- Billing cards (manual, nearly obsolete and carry a penalty)
- Machine readable input/output
- Physical media:
  - Discs 3½" Mac or IBM.
  - Magnetic tape (used by larger facilities)
  - 380 IBM cartridge
- Electronic data transfer (EDT); sent by modem
- Claims will be returned in the same format in which you send them. E.g., If you submit claims by magnetic tape, your reports will be sent back by tape.

Timelines

- Claims must be in by the 18th of every month to be guaranteed payment within that cycle.
- If you use EDT you can send in claims up to the end of the month, and they will be paid if the claims office is not too busy.
- Payment is by the 18th of the next month.

Information Components
(Many of these data are entered automatically on some software programs but must be entered manually on cards.)

Client's demographic data

- Full name
- Address
- Date of birth
- Gender
- Province or territory

Additional card information
- Health card number
- Version code, if applicable
- Expiry date (on some systems)

Provider number

Payment program (most computers default to HCP)

Payee (who is getting the money: P for provider and S for client; opted-out only; rarely used)

Accounting number (usually computer-generated; optional)

Date of service

Service code, procedural code, or both

PPU (price per unit/service)

Number of services (may appear on screen as units)

Diagnostic code fee (the same as PPU unless service is time based or more than one service is claimed)

Facility number, used only if the client has been admitted to a hospital or other facility

Referring number, used only if the claim is by a specialist; the referring physician's registration number

Admission date, used only for a client in hospital

SLI STABILITY LIFE INSURANCE COMPANY

PO Box 12345
Edmonton, AB
T3G 5N6
780-564-2929

Consent for Release of Information

I authorize the Stability Life Insurance Company to conduct a thorough medical assessment for my condition and:

1. to be allowed to receive, review, and obtain copies of all hospital, medical, X-ray, laboratory, psychological, vocational and other related records related to my medical condition that will assist in completing this assessment and

2. to discuss any relevant information including test results or identifying information with the appropriate health professionals, employer, or related insurance personnel involved in my assessment, disability, and/or rehabilitation process.

I agree to the appropriate photocopying of this information as deemed necessary by those involved in my assessment.

I understand that the main purpose of this referral and gathering of information is for the purpose of assessing my medical condition and determining my entitlement to the appropriate benefits and/or rehabilitation.

DATED THIS 2ND DAY OF JANUARY 2004

At Edmonton, Alberta

SIGNATURE *John Doe*

WITNESS *JR Benesh*

Figure 12.10 Consent form for release of information to insurance company.

Summary

1. Claims submission is one of your major responsibilities. Claims submission is a complex process that has been simplified by the use of specially designed computer software. You need a solid understanding of codes. Focus on accuracy since errors can result in rejected claims.

2. Claims may be submitted on tape or disk or by electronic data transfer (EDT). Some provinces will still accept submission on billing cards but penalize the few providers who still use them. EDT is becoming the most widely used method because it is the most efficient. It also improves cash flow by allowing faster response to submissions and payment of submissions later in the billing period.

3. When registering a client, it is important to verify client information. Health card validation reduces claims rejection and facilitates prompt claims payment.

4. A variety of software programs are available to facilitate claims preparation. Common modules include registration, billing day sheets, and billing modules. Software can integrate clients' personal and medical information with billing records.

5. A claim must include certain information: physician registration number, client demographic data, payment program, service date, service code, diagnostic code (usually), number of services, price per unit, and fee. Claims may be flagged for independent consideration, and explanations can be added in a manual review field.

6. With the exception of certain excluded services, reciprocal medical billing is handled like a regular claim except that the payment program is RMB. In Ontario, as well as some other provinces, the Ministry of Health acts as the payment agency for most workers' compensation claims. Be sure to identify the payment program as WCB (or WSIB).

7. Reports from the ministry in response to claims submissions are supplied in the same format in which the claims are submitted. These reports include remittance advice reports, claims error reports, and, for EDT, file reject messages and batch edit reports.

8. Review claims error reports and resubmit claims. Review the next RA form to see whether resubmitted claims have been paid. If a claim is rejected again, submit an RA inquiry.

9. A range of services are not covered by provincial/territorial health-care plans and are chargeable directly to clients. Clients must be told before the service is provided how much it will cost. Some physicians offer block or annual fees rather than charging for individual services. Most physicians ask for payment at the time of service. Firmness prevents problems with outstanding accounts.

10. Third-party services are those done at the request of someone other than the client. Third parties include government agencies, employers, schools, and insurance companies. Insurance companies often require examinations, medical information, and a variety of forms to be filled out. Doctors may also be asked to testify in court.

Key Terms

ELECTRONIC DATA TRANSFER (EDT) **320**	MACHINE-READABLE INPUT (MRI) **320** PARTIAL CLAIMS PAYMENTS **334**	REMITTANCE ADVICE (RA) **333** THIRD-PARTY SERVICE **337**

Review Questions

1. Outline, in sequence, the steps of the client registration process.

2. List three methods of submitting health insurance claims.

3. What are the main advantages of electronic data transfer?

4. What is the purpose of the accounting number used in claims submission?

5. List and explain the payment programs used in claims submission.

6. What is the manual review field on a billing screen used for?

7. State the difference between a batch edit report and a file edit report.

8. Describe the purpose and content of a remittance advice report.

9. What should you do when you receive a claims error report?

10. Explain each of the headings in the following screen sample:

ITEM CODE	PPU	Units	Type	Date	Diag. Code	MR	Amount	Status

Application Exercises

1. Compare the advantages and disadvantages of electronic claims submission versus submission on disk or tape.

2. Research electronic claims submission in your province or territory. Identify the files generated by this electronic billing system. Compare them with those described in this chapter, considering name, purpose, and content. Are claims submission deadlines the same as those discussed in this chapter?

3. For each of the following scenarios, fill in all the applicable fields in the chart representing the billing screen. Current amounts can be obtained from your province's health plan billing schedule Web site.

   a. Ivy comes in to have her ears syringed.

   b. Mia comes in for some family planning advice. She is worried about the risks of becoming pregnant. The doctor spends time counselling Mia about genetic risk factors. Mia also has a Pap smear while she is in.

   c. Craig comes in complaining of vague symptoms of diarrhea and epigastric discomfort. The doctor does a fairly thorough examination, but cannot reach a conclusive diagnosis.

   d. Dr. Shymloski has seen Peter several times for a complaint of chest tightness. He sends Peter to Dr. Jamison, an internist, for a consultation. You work for Dr. Shymloski.

   e. Complete the chart for the scenario in part d. This time you work for Dr. Jamison.

   f. Dr. Oran made a house call for Mrs. Erickson at 9:30 p.m. Her diagnosis was congestive heart failure.

   g. Regina was assessed for complications of her diabetes, and her insulin regimen was regulated. Home care was ordered to assess and apply a dressing to her foot.

   h. At 1 a.m., the doctor delivered Tina Smalley's baby. It was a spontaneous delivery with no complications.

   i. The doctor is unable to make a diagnosis for Meena and has put on the chart that she has a collection of vague symptoms.

   j. Lana's diagnosis was a plantar wart. The doctor removed the wart using a chemical substance.

To those familiar with a highly sophisticated health information environment, some of these methods may seem somewhat archaic. However, they do work, and they are relatively commonplace. The methods used for chart identification and retrieval reflect those choices discussed earlier.

Alphabetical

Alphabetical filing is one of the oldest and most straightforward systems. Alphabetical filing systems do not require an index. They are considered direct access systems because you need only have the client's name to file or find the record. However, they require the user to be a reasonably good speller.

Using this system, last names are used first, followed by the first name, and then the second name, if applicable. Names are filed by the first different letter. For example, Reid comes before Sachs; Sachs comes before Smith; Smith comes before Smyth; Smyth comes before Smythe. Use legal names, not nicknames or short forms; thus, Robert Smith would come after Richard Smith even if Robert is usually called Bob.

Alphabetical order works well if there is no opportunity of misspelling a client's name. However, even if the client has been registered with the correct spelling and the record is correctly filed, looking for the name under a misspelling may make it hard to find the record.

To overcome problems with misspelling, some organizations use a filing technique known as *phonetic* or *soundex* filing. This method groups similar-sounding consonants together and removes all vowels. While this has largely gone out of vogue in paper-based systems because it is complex and not easily learned, computer-based registration systems use algorithms to search for names phonetically. Some systems group all names beginning with Mc and Mac together at the beginning (or at the end) of the M section.

In a family practice, if members of a family have different surnames, charts may be cross-referenced.

Numeric

Numeric filing systems are effective with records that are filed and retrieved by number. Unfortunately, filing systems that are organized by a strict numeric sequence almost always require an index or pointer to the record location. If client records are asked for by name, you would need an index that would give the number for each name. For this reason, numeric systems that require an index are sometimes called *indirect access systems*.

There are two methods of filing numbered records: straight numeric and terminal digit.

STRAIGHT NUMERIC Sometimes called a consecutive numeric system, this system files consecutively numbered files or documents in a strict sequential order (i.e., 101, 102, 103, etc.). As an example, medical records 123455, 123456, and 123457 would all be filed side by side. This system is normally used for records that are prenumbered, such as cheques, invoices, vouchers, and purchase orders. This method of filing requires very little training.

TERMINAL DIGIT Terminal-digit filing is a variation of straight numeric and was developed to overcome congestion in large filing systems when the most active records are being filed in consecutive order. (This is not usually a concern in an office; these systems are mostly used in large facilities.) Basing the filing sequence on the last few digits of the number disperses the files throughout the system, thus allowing easier access. Terminal digit is particularly valuable when dealing with a long number string. This system segments a number into component parts. As an example, number 123456 could be broken into three segments: 12-34-56. Reading the segments right to left, 56 is the terminal digit, 34 is the secondary digit, and 12 is the primary digit. In this example, the total filing area would be partitioned into 100 filing sections (00–99). Each section would be partitioned into 100 areas, and each area would have room for 100 records. Record 12-34-56 would be filed in section 56, area 34, and would be record 12. Records 11-34-55 and 13-34-57 would be filed immediately before and after record 12-34-56. Middle digit and primary digit filing are variations of the terminal digit sequencing.

Colour Coding

Some practices combine either the alphabetical or numeric method of filing with colour coding. The file folders themselves can be different colours, or you can buy coloured tabs to add to neutral-coloured file folders. Each letter in the alphabet, or each number, may have a specific colour. In a busy office with a large number of charts, colour coding can prevent misfiling (because a misplaced file will stand out) and make it faster to find a chart.

Centralized versus Decentralized Storage

PURGE   (of file) review and reorganize to remove outdated or irrelevant information.

Record storage may be centralized or decentralized. Private practices use a centralized system: all records are stored in one location until they are **purged**. Hospitals may use centralized, decentralized, or a combination thereof, depending on the facilities' policies, size, geographic proximity to treatment areas, record sensitivity, and staff availability.

CENTRALIZED Centralized filing systems designate one location in which to house all records. In a hospital, this is usually the Health Records Department. All health information on a particular patient is stored in one physical chart and is located in one department.

DECENTRALIZED Decentralized filing systems allow parts of the patient record to reside in areas outside the central Health Records Department, although the locations of these parts of the record are available through the MPI. Records that would not be needed for all visits may be stored in specific clinics, such as ophthalmology, audiology, and dental clinics. This can be convenient if the hospital is spread over more than one site. Particularly sensitive records, such as those relating to therapeutic abortion or AIDS, may also be kept in the treatment areas to keep them out of general circulation.

Filing Equipment

The File Folder

Regardless of the method of organizing files, most agencies and providers keep paper files in file folders. These are cardboard folders that come in a variety of colours, thicknesses, and finishes. The two most popular sizes are standard and legal. If you use cabinets, putting the regular file folders inside hanging folders makes them easier to retrieve.

Storage Systems

A variety of filing equipment is available, from open-faced stacks to lockable cabinets, from static shelving to mobile files. Choice of filing equipment is generally driven by space and accessibility.

Shelves

Filing shelves are commonly used in doctors' offices because the charts are visible and easily accessible. For high shelves, you may need a step stool to retrieve files from the top shelves, which saves space but takes time. The charts are stored horizontally along each shelf. Some shelves have doors or covers that can be locked. If the shelves are open, they must be in an area that can be properly secured. Figure 13.5 shows traditional shelving. Even more space saving is mobile shelving, shown in Figure 13.6, in which one layer of shelving slides in front of another, allowing almost twice as many files to fit on a wall.

Filing Cabinets

Filing cabinets may be vertical or horizontal. They may be moved and stacked and usually have fronts that can be closed and locked for security reasons. Filing cabinets often do not afford maximum filing capacity for limited space.

The decision to choose a vertical file or a lateral file depends on what kind of room it is going into. If you have more wall space than floor space, a lateral file is generally your best bet. If wall space is at a premium, but floor space is more readily available, then vertical files would probably meet your needs more effectively.

A third choice is circular filing cabinets (also called rotary filing cabinets). Figure 13.7 shows a file storage system that is a cabinet within a cabinet. The interior is a four-sided storage cabinet that revolves completely in either direction with only a touch; you can turn it like a lazy Susan to reach the file you need. Circular files are a reasonable choice for practices where space is limited but do not usually hold many files. They are sometimes used in nursing stations in health-care facilities.

The term rotary file or circular file is also used for a small filing box that can sit on the top of your desk (also commonly known by the brand name Rolodex). This file is divided alphabetically and is useful for entering frequently used names, numbers, addresses, and Web sites, such as those for physicians to which your practice commonly refers clients, drug stores, suppliers of office stationery, laboratories, and community agencies.

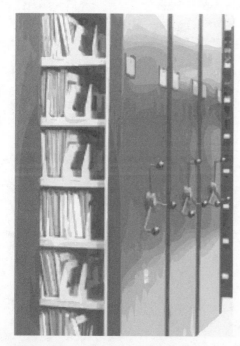

Figure 13.5 Traditional shelving.

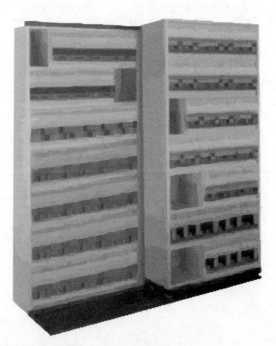

Figure 13.6 Mobile shelving.

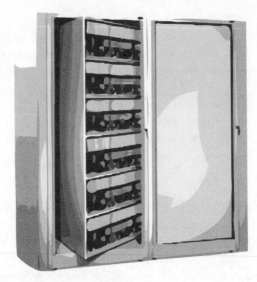

Figure 13.7 Circular or rotary filing cabinet.

Temporary Filing Space

You will often have a few files pulled for reference. Perhaps you are holding the file for the physician to look at in reviewing a medication renewal request, or you are waiting for a report to add to the file. Some people keep a stack of such files on their desks or loose on a shelf. However, it is all too easy for someone picking something up from your desk to inadvertently scoop up one of these files as well. It can then end up sitting on the bottom of a pile of papers, or misfiled, leading to frustration and wasted time. It is better to have a special place to keep such files, called "**auxiliary files**." This could be a drawer of a filing cabinet or a desktop device such as an expanding file, a set of trays, an incline sorter, or a hanging file rack. The rack can be divided into sections for reports, medication renewal, outgoing call information, and so on. As soon as you are finished with the file, return it promptly to its proper place.

AUXILIARY FILE a temporary filing space for files in current use.

Filing Office Forms

Even offices that keep client records on computer will have some papers to file. For example, every office has a number of blank forms and documents, some of which are used more frequently than others. The most efficient method of filing this type of thing is by subject. Variations on this method exist, some very creative. Some systems incorporate alphabetical or alphanumeric sorting and colour coding. For subject filing, it is a good idea to have a broad subject category followed by more specific categories. For example:

Insurance Forms
    State Farm
    Sun Life
    WSIB

Requisitions
    Biochemistry
    Hematology
    MRI
    Ultrasound
    Upper GI

CHAPTER 14

The Hospital Setting

On completing this chapter, you will be able to:

1. List the types of health-care facilities.
2. Discuss the concept and purpose of hospital accreditation.
3. Outline the typical organizational structure of a hospital.
4. Summarize the types of hospital restructuring taking place in Canada.
5. List the departments found in hospitals and discuss the purpose of each.
6. List the responsibilities of the various types of health professionals in the hospital setting.
7. Identify the responsibilities of the clinical secretary.
8. Describe the components of a client-care unit.
9. Summarize the functions of computers in hospitals.
10. Apply the principles of confidentiality in the hospital environment.
11. Discuss hospital security.

A hospital is a health-care facility that is licensed by the province or territory to provide a range of health-care services on both inpatient and outpatient bases. Hospitals' basic functions include

◆ providing expert medical, surgical, or psychiatric diagnosis and care;
◆ preventing disease and promoting health;
◆ meeting the needs of their communities (with input from district health organizations); and
◆ conducting health-related research and education.

This chapter outlines the structure and functions of a hospital, the various hospital departments, and the responsibilities of a clinical secretary. Health office professionals in hospitals and clinics may also be called ward clerks or health unit coordinators, but clinical secretary is one of the more common terms, and it will be used throughout this part of the book.

The responsibilities are tremendous, the pace in most areas is fast, and stress is part of the job, yet working in the hospital environment is both exciting and rewarding.

Kinds of Health-Care Facilities

Most health-care facilities in Canada are publicly operated and funded by the provincial or federal government, although some private, for-profit facilities do exist across the country. "Private" does not necessarily mean that clients pay for services. The province may pay private facilities a fee to provide medically necessary services. Clients receiving insured services present their health cards, and doctors performing these services bill the provincial/territorial plan just as they would in a public hospital. These facilities may also offer uninsured or enhanced services, which clients would pay for (as discussed in Chapter 10). Such facilities are a bit of an anomaly in most provinces, and many Canadians have reservations about any increase in privately operated facilities, seeing it as a step away from public health care.

There are several classifications of health-care facilities, some of which are province specific. The most common are

- general or acute care hospitals (may include specialty hospitals, such as the Hospital for Sick Children in Toronto);
- convalescent hospitals;
- chronic care hospitals;
- nursing homes;
- active treatment/teaching psychiatric hospitals; and
- active treatment facilities for alcohol and drug addiction (rehabilitation hospitals, federal hospitals).

General Hospitals

ACUTE CARE   care for a client who is acutely ill, that is, very ill, but with an illness expected to run a short course, (as opposed to a chronic illness). Acute care is provided for clients with a variety of health problems.

A general hospital provides the community with a variety of services, 24 hours day, seven days a week, ranging from medical/surgical to obstetric and psychiatric services, both on inpatient and outpatient bases. This type of hospital may also be referred to as an **acute care** hospital because the majority of hospital beds are designated for those with acute illnesses and conditions. However, they may also have beds designated for chronic care, rehabilitation, palliative care, and respite care. Chronic care beds are usually for short terms, and clients needing long-term care are transferred to a chronic care institute. The kinds and levels of care available vary. Teaching hospitals also provide learning opportunities for medical students.

Convalescent Hospitals

A convalescent hospital provides recuperative care to individuals who are expected to recover and return to their own homes or to other community placements. A physician and skilled nursing staff are available round the clock.

Chronic Care Facilities

CHRONIC CARE   care for someone with a chronic illness, that is, one that typically progresses slowly but lasts for a long time, often lifelong.

A **chronic care** facility provides long-term inpatient medical care for people with little or no potential for rehabilitation. Clients may have chronic illnesses, such as multiple sclerosis, advanced chronic obstructive pulmonary disease (COPD), or some dementias. Other clients may have severe physical disabilities that require hospital treatment, may have suffered a head or spinal cord injury, or may be past the acute phase of treatment but require ongoing hospital care.

Nursing Homes

Nursing homes provide continuous nursing and medical care for individuals who cannot be maintained at home and who are chronically ill and/or incapacitated. They do not, however, have all the facilities of an acute care hospital. People in a nursing home depend on the staff for such activities as dressing, walking, bathing, and sometimes feeding. (In contrast, retirement homes are essentially housing choices for individuals capable of living in a reasonably independent manner but which may provide a range of supportive services that are either included in the fee or that are purchased separately.) These may be either publicly or privately funded. Clients at a private facility pay the full cost; for public facilities, government subsidies are available to clients who need them. Some provinces offer an income tax break for clients paying for retirement accommodation.

Rehabilitation Hospitals

Rehabilitation hospitals are for people needing professional assistance to restore physical functioning following an illness, injury, or surgery.

Psychiatric Hospitals

A psychiatric hospital provides diagnosis and intensive and continued clinical therapy for mental illness and mental rehabilitation. (Many general hospitals also offer psychiatric inpatient and outpatient services.)

Drug Addiction/Alcoholic Treatment Centres

These facilities can be publicly or privately funded and offer rehabilitative care for those suffering from drug and/or alcohol addiction. Most facilities have follow-up programs that offer treatment, guidance, and support to clients after discharge.

Federal Hospitals

Federal hospitals are operated throughout Canada by departments of the federal government for the care of special groups of patients. Included are such facilities as military hospitals, veterans' homes, and hospitals for First Nations people.

Hospitals may also be categorized by size and type of service offered. A *primary care* hospital offers basic care, including health promotion and prevention of illness. It is mainly community based. A secondary care hospital offers specialist services. A tertiary care hospital offers highly specialized skills, technology, and support services for clients with acute and chronic illnesses. This type of hospital is usually found in a big city and often takes clients referred from smaller hospitals.

Accreditation of Health-Care Facilities

Standards for excellence in health-care facilities across Canada are maintained by a periodic assessment of each facility by the Canadian Council of Health Services Accreditation (CCHSA). Although obtaining CCHSA accreditation is voluntary, most organizations opt for it because it enhances their status. Formal accreditation assessments occur about every three years and give the organization an overview of its strengths and the areas where it can improve. The CCHSA looks at how the organization compares with national standards in the following areas:

◆ Quality of care
◆ Community accessibility
◆ Appropriateness of care (i.e., does the intervention meet the client's needs?)
◆ Effectiveness of care

- ◆ Timeliness
- ◆ Continuity of care (i.e., Are clients followed up? Is care modified, if needed? For example, if a client comes to a diabetic clinic for teaching, does the facility follow through until the client has met the learning goals?)
- ◆ Safety

If the organization meets all of the standards, it becomes an accredited organization, usually for another three years. If a facility falls short, it may be accredited for a year, during which time it is expected to correct the areas in which it was deficient. Losing accreditation not only undermines the facility's reputation but it can also lose its funding.

The period leading up to accreditation is hectic and stressful in any organization. Most organizations conduct their own review to prepare for the formal assessment. Every component of every service and procedure, both clinical and administrative, is put under a microscope. The goal is to maintain and improve adherence to all standards at all times. This is not entirely realistic. As a clinical secretary, you will be heavily involved in the administrative components of review and evaluation. The work can be overwhelming. The process can be made bearable if everyone involved is organized, efficient, and works as a team.

The Organizational Structure of a Hospital

Except for the few privately run ones, hospitals are nonprofit corporations that operate under a special section of the *Corporations Act*, which is provincial legislation. Rules, regulations, and corporate structures vary by province or territory. Most of these hospitals have formed partnerships with other hospitals/organizations, resulting in centralized management.

As corporations, hospitals are headed by a board of directors. The board of directors is, in theory, elected by its membership. What constitutes the hospital membership varies across Canada. Members may include donors and interested community members. Board members are elected for specific terms; they may be re-elected. Each board will have a nominating committee that accepts nominations of members of the community or invites members to consider standing for election.

The board of directors appoints a chief executive officer (CEO) for their hospital or partnership of hospitals. The CEO is a salaried position, and the CEO is accountable to the board of directors. The CEO is ultimately responsible for the management of the organization, including such things as hiring and operating within a budget set by the board of directors.

The remaining organizational structure of each hospital will be different but will follow similar guidelines. There may be several vice-presidents or vice-chairs reporting to the CEO, chair, or president; in some structures, vice-presidents may report to an executive vice-president. A hospital involved in a **collaborative partnership** usually has a site administrator or a clinical administrator who oversees the daily operation of the hospital. Most hospitals also have a chief of staff who represents the hospital's medical staff. There will be someone who is responsible for each department or group of departments within the organization, such as chief of medicine, chief of surgery, manager of information technology, and director of acute care services. Titles and exact responsibilities of positions vary among hospitals and may shift rapidly within a hospital. Generally, the position of clinical leader or clinical manager has replaced that of

COLLABORATIVE PARTNERSHIP the relationship among hospitals that have entered into an agreement to form a partnership, sharing clinical and administrative responsibilities.

worker draws on community resources to meet the client's needs. If the client cannot return home, a social worker will work with the client and family to find an alternative solution, such as placement in a long-term care facility. Social workers also provide clients with support and counselling.

The Professional Staff

If you work in a hospital, you will interact with many different health-care professionals. Each type of facility will have a somewhat different mix. For example, a nursing home will have proportionally fewer registered nurses (RNs) than a hospital and more registered practical nurses (RPNs) and personal support workers.

It is important to know who these professionals are and how they contribute to the health team. In reading the following section, keep in mind that titles and job descriptions vary with facility and location and are constantly shifting as facilities try to improve efficiency while following trends in political correctness.

Physicians

As discussed in Chapter 4, some physicians are salaried and on staff full time at hospitals, especially teaching hospitals. Emergentologists may work only at a hospital; they may be salaried or bill fee-for-service. Many doctors, including general practitioners and specialists such as internists and cardiologists, have private practices outside the hospital; they attend their own clients in hospital. Surgeons may be salaried to work in a hospital but also have private practices. Anesthetists work almost exclusively in hospitals but usually bill fee-for-service.

Health-care providers, such as physicians and midwives, must apply to a hospital for admitting privileges before they can admit clients to that facility and actively participate in the client's treatment. In a process called **credentialling**, their qualifications are first carefully examined by a committee composed of members of the medical staff and perhaps someone from the hospital administration. The provider must then follow the facility's policies and regulations and may have admitting privileges revoked if she fails to meet standards of conduct, practice, and care.

CREDENTIALLING a process whereby a peer group judges an individual's qualifications to perform certain services.

Unit Manager or Clinical Leader

In the traditional hospital structure, each hospital unit was typically managed by a head nurse. The head nurse almost always worked on the day shift. She did not routinely provide patient care but oversaw all activities that took place on the floor and acted as the primary contact for physicians. She would accompany doctors on their rounds to visit clients, often writing down the physicians' orders. She was a fount of information on each client's condition and treatment plan. She also reviewed all clients' medications for the day and checked the charts for any missed orders. Unless absent from the client-care unit, the head nurse transcribed all doctors' orders. She completed a staffing schedule for each day and assigned a charge nurse for each shift. Other nurses on the floor would take direction from the charge nurse.

Today, a nurse does not usually accompany the physician on rounds. Instead of instructing a nurse, the doctor writes down the orders or enters them directly into the computer at the bedside using a portable device (discussed in Chapter 16) and informs the client's nurse about anything critical. Each client-care unit still has a person who is ultimately responsible for the unit, as well as someone on each shift who takes a lead role. Nursing staff and the clinical secretary first turn to this shift leader if they have problems and then to the unit manager.

The person responsible for the unit may be called a *manager* or *clinical leader*. This person may or may not be a nurse. She may be responsible for several floors or units, usually related ones; for example, she may be manager of Surgical and Emergency Services or of Inpatient Medical Services. This person is still usually the ultimate reporting authority for the clinical secretary.

The Clinical Resource Nurse

The person who coordinates and manages a unit for a shift is still sometimes called a charge nurse but is more often called a clinical resource nurse; other titles also exist. This person is always a nurse but may be on a full-time or part-time basis. One person may be permanently assigned to a shift, or several people with the same title may rotate through shifts. This is the person you will work most closely with, who will check your processed doctors' orders, and to whom you will take any problems that arise during the course of your shift.

Nursing Staff

Each unit will have different nursing requirements. Some units, such as the Intensive Care Unit (ICU), use only RNs. Although some hospitals hire only RNs, in most hospitals, other units also employ RPNs and sometimes health-care aides or personal support workers (PSWs). Some units use team nursing. A team may consist of one RN and two RPNs (or sometimes two RNs and one RPN). The RN is the team leader.

Registered Nurses

The College of Nurses in each province clearly outlines nursing responsibilities of each level of nurse. An RN may be a graduate of a diploma or a degree program, usually of three or four years. (Ontario has phased out diploma programs in favour of BScN degrees.) After graduation and before writing provincial examinations, the nurse is known as a *graduate nurse*. Upon successful completion of provincial examinations, he becomes a registered nurse. Qualifications are specific to the province or territory; an RN who moves from Ontario to British Columbia or Newfoundland will have to recertify by taking that province's exams. Usually, RNs are the only nurses who may dispense medications; they maintain responsibility for the drug cart. RNs are also the only nurses who can carry out delegated responsibilities, such as giving intravenous medications, looking after acutely ill clients, monitoring patient-controlled analgesic pumps, doing complex dressings, and inserting nasogastric tubes.

Registered Practical Nurses

The RPN is a graduate of a college program that varies from one-and-a-half to two years in length. These practitioners used to be called registered nurses' assistants (RNA), but the title was changed to more accurately reflect their status as independent health-care professionals. The scope of practice of the RPN is more limited than that of the RN, although it has expanded greatly in recent years. For example, although RPNs do not normally give out medications in acute care settings, they do in nursing homes and chronic care hospitals.

Personal Support Workers

This position used to be called a health-care aide, but the term *personal support worker* (PSW) is becoming more popular in some regions. Some agencies still train PSWs on the job, but most are graduates of a three- to six-month certificate program at a community college or equivalent. Although some PSWs work as team members with nurses in hospitals, they are more likely to work in nursing homes, long-term care facilities, and community agencies.

Orderlies

Some hospitals employ orderlies (usually male) to carry out such duties as transporting clients. They may be trained to bathe clients and perform such tasks as male catheterization, especially when there is no male nurse available and a client is uncomfortable with being treated by a woman. Orderlies may be trained on the job.

Housekeeping Staff

Housekeeping staff are often assigned to specific units, although they may rotate. Among their duties are cleaning and disinfecting vacated beds and bedside accessories. You may be responsible for notifying housekeeping (often electronically) when a client has been discharged so that they can clean the room. It is important to communicate clearly with the housekeeping staff to ensure efficient use of hospital beds. Some clinical secretaries keep an updated list of discharges on the floor for housekeeping staff to refer to (often a book kept at the desk in the nurses' station). There may be times when a bed is urgently needed, but a discharged client is still occupying it. If the client is able, he may be asked to wait in the reception area so that the bed can be prepared for the new admission.

Most hospitals request that discharged clients leave by a certain time, often 11 a.m. Do your best to encourage the client to leave on time to allow for the room to be prepared. Often, elective (nonemergency) admissions are asked to come in around 3 p.m.

Pharmacists

Many client-care units have an assigned pharmacist and/or pharmacy assistant. Pharmacists are university graduates, often entering into pharmacy with an undergraduate degree in the sciences (see Chapter 7). Among other things, the pharmacist manages the stocking of medications, often for more than one floor.

Physiotherapists

Physiotherapists are university graduates, often with an undergraduate degree in kinesiology and a master's in physiotherapy. If you process an order for physiotherapy, you would phone or e-mail the Physiotherapy Department. If a client is ambulatory, she will probably go to the Physiotherapy Department; if not, the physiotherapist will come to the client. Note the appointment time on the kardex or client intervention screen. Keep a list of the client's activities to avoid scheduling conflicts and ensure that the client is ready. For example, if Jovana (who relies on the nurses to help her get bathed and up in the morning) has an 8.30 a.m. appointment with the physiotherapist, make a note so that the nurse can plan to get her ready on time.

Respiratory Therapists

A respiratory therapist (RT) may be a graduate of a three- or four-year college program or may have a master's degree. RTs provide inhalation treatments, set up and monitor oxygen therapy, manage clients on respirators or using spirometers, obtain blood gases, and monitor clients' respiratory progress. There is usually an RT covering all shifts, and one will respond to a cardiac or a respiratory arrest. Nurses will initiate oxygen therapy if an RT is unavailable.

Laboratory Technologists and Technicians

Medical laboratory technologists, as discussed in Chapter 6, are graduates of a post-secondary program and perform a vast array of laboratory tests ordered by the doctor, with the help of laboratory technicians and sometimes phlebotomists.

Dietitians

Registered dietitians are university graduates, usually from a four-year program. They may be helped by dietary assistants. You will work with dietitians and dietary assistants when arranging dietary counselling, processing nutritional orders, or cancelling or delaying a client's meal because of tests.

Responsibilities of the Clinical Secretary

CLINICAL SECRETARY (SC) or WARD CLERK   a health office professional working in a hospital; an individual who assumes responsibilities for the secretarial, clerical, communication, and other designated needs of a hospital unit or department.

The **clinical secretary** is often described as the hub in the wheel that keeps the client-care unit operational. Consider the following comments by nurses:

"If our clinical secretary calls in sick, I get a sinking feeling in my stomach. We can't really manage without her."

"Our clinical secretary holds our floor together."

"The clinical secretary on our unit is the best thing that ever happened to us. She is competent, organized, and keeps everything on track and running smoothly."

"We simply would not be able to manage without our clinical secretary. I sometimes wonder how she keeps up with the doctors' orders and also keeps our unit so organized."

The scope of responsibilities and duties discussed here is general. Exactly how you carry out these duties will depend on the type of client-care unit, the facility's policies and organization, and how computerized the hospital is.

Clerical/Secretarial Responsibilities

If you work on a client-care unit, you will likely

- manage the administrative components of admission, discharge, and transfer;
- prepare and update identity bracelets, bed labels, and so on;
- orient new admissions to the unit;
- distribute client mail;
- transcribe orders accurately and promptly (see Chapter 16);
- notify nurses of stat orders and changes in clients' care;
- keep charts up-to-date and prepare forms;
- label charts with client information and doctor's name;
- ensure that requisitions for blood work, specimens, and X-rays are completed and recorded;
- ensure that lab results are recorded and directed appropriately;
- update unit forms and policy and procedure manuals;
- maintain staffing schedules;
- enter data for client care hours/workload analysis;

The same rules apply to in-person conversations. Any medical information about a client must remain confidential. Some people may think that sharing good news is harmless, but that is no excuse to breach confidentiality. Consider the following situation:

A student we will call Jane was working in labour and delivery when a family friend came in and delivered a baby girl. The student went across to the residence to get a book and then went back to the delivery room. As she passed the hall telephone, Rebecca, another student nurse and a mutual friend, shouted out, "Jane . . . I hear Elisabeth had her baby. . . What did she have?" "A girl," replied Jane breathlessly as she rushed back to the hospital. Rebecca made a few phone calls. By the time Elisabeth's husband got out of the delivery room and phoned her parents to announce the new arrival, they already knew. He felt robbed of the opportunity of sharing the news firsthand. This was a blatant breach of confidentiality on the part of both student nurses.

Be mindful of confidentiality at all times, and do not release any information without the client's express consent.

Security

Security is a concern in any hospital and becomes more complex in a larger and busier environment. Since the devastating events of September 11, 2001, and the subsequent anthrax attacks in the United States, facilities across the continent have begun to review their emergency planning. Very few facilities would be truly prepared to cope with a bioterrorist attack. Yet hospitals now consider themselves potential targets and are upgrading disaster plans to deal with types of attack that still seem unthinkable. They should be able to respond promptly and effectively to an internal threat and to meet the needs of the community in the event of a widespread threat or disaster. This includes being adequately stocked with antibiotics, antitoxins, antidotes, and other emergency equipment needed to treat and sustain potential victims. Hospital laboratories in many larger hospitals are moving to improve their technology for prompt identification of potentially infectious substances. Response to potential bioterrorist attacks should be incorporated into the training and drills for hospital staff.

Although the risk of a terrorist attack is low in most Canadian communities, disasters, such as flood, fire, or violence, can strike without warning. Consider the effects of the forest fires that ravaged British Columbia in the summer of 2003. Most communities see hospitals as a critical resource for medical management of any external disaster. Links with other health facilities and community emergency resources are essential if a hospital is to respond efficiently. Every staff member must have a role and be prepared to perform it efficiently. You may be asked to assist in organizing client evacuation, triaging clients, recording events, or managing the communication centre. You may be on a reserve list to be called in if such a disaster occurs. You may be calling others in should the need arise. You can prepare to do your share in the event of a disaster by knowing your role, attending in-service seminars, and participating in any mock disaster drills.

Security and Emergency Codes

Even without terrorist attacks or community-wide disasters, hospitals by their nature are subject to a daily risk of smaller-scale emergencies. All hospitals use a set of "universal codes" to alert staff to a variety of emergencies. The codes in Table 14.1 are those recommended by the Ontario Hospital Association; other provinces may use different codes.

Table 14.1 | Universal Emergency Codes (Ontario)

Code	Emergency
Red	Fire
White	Violent client or physical danger
Green	Evacuation
Orange	External disaster
Brown	Internal chemical spill
Blue	Cardiac arrest
Pink	Pediatric cardiac arrest
Yellow	Missing client
Black	Bomb threat

It may be your responsibility to give the emergency signal.

◆ Know the protocol. Know your role.

◆ Stay calm; getting upset will only impede your ability to respond.

◆ Get all the information needed (including the location of the emergency), and make sure it is accurate.

◆ Promptly notify the appropriate persons.

In many hospitals, you would notify switchboard or the central communications operator. For example, in the event of a cardiac arrest, you may be required to dial switchboard and say, "Code blue in room 342, west three south."

Missing Clients

Sometimes, a client will go missing—most often a confused or disoriented client. Such a client is at risk, particularly if she requires urgent or continuous medical care. There are also times when clients will simply walk out for personal reasons, for example, if they are dissatisfied with the medical care they are receiving (or not receiving). As soon as you hear that a client seems to be missing, initiate a search. If you learn that the client has left the unit, announce the appropriate code to notify staff. Internal guidelines will spell out how staff are given further information, such as a description of the client. Security will participate in the search inside the hospital and on hospital grounds. If the client cannot be located promptly, the police will be notified to assist with a broader search.

If a client threatens to walk out of the hospital, try to locate a nurse or physician to reason with him. If the client is upset enough to try leaving, there may be no reasoning. If he refuses to wait or to discuss his concerns, ask him to sign a waiver stating that he has left the hospital without permission of the provider and assumes full responsibility for his own health status. Some will sign, and some will refuse. If he refuses, note down the fact and the time of departure.

Identification Tags

Most facilities require all personnel to wear photo ID tags. If someone you do not know comes to your unit without proper identification, introduce yourself, ask if you can help, and ask for his name and professional designation. For all you know, he may be the hospital's chief of staff—but err on the side of caution. If the person acts suspicious, aggressive, or argumentative or refuses to identify himself, get help. Do not confront anyone alone if you feel the situation is potentially volatile or dangerous.

Secure Units

Some areas may be designated secure units. The psychiatric unit may be one and the maternal/child unit another. Just how secure these units are and what type of security they have may vary. Often, they have a camera to show anyone who is approaching. Some units may be locked, and designated staff will have keys. There will be a bell or signal at the door, which the approaching individual will activate. It may be your responsibility to open the door. If you do not recognize the person, ask for identification and the purpose for visiting the unit. There may be individuals who are not welcome in the unit. For example, a new mother may have told staff that she does not want to see her estranged partner. Follow agency protocol when handling such situations. Intensive care units, although not usually designated secure, will also have restrictions on who may visit and when. Visitors are often required to ring a bell; a nurse will answer and determine whether it is in the client's interest to have a visitor at that moment.

Summary

1. Working in a hospital is challenging, at times stressful, but rewarding. To function competently as a clinical secretary, you must have effective organizational, communication, and computer skills and be able to interact adaptively with a wide range of clients and professionals.

2. Health-care facilities include general (primarily acute care) hospitals, convalescent hospitals, chronic care facilities, nursing homes, rehabilitation hospitals, psychiatric hospitals, and drug addiction/alcohol treatment centres. Accreditation, while not mandatory, enhances status and funding opportunities. Preparing for accreditation is a hectic process.

3. Hospitals are managed by a board of directors, in most cases, elected, and by a salaried CEO. Most hospitals are in partnerships with a central management. Nursing staff include registered nurses, registered practical nurses, and, sometimes, personal support workers. The clinical secretary often reports to the clinical resource nurse (or charge nurse) and ultimately to a clinical leader or unit manager.

4. Almost all departments are interdependent in some manner. Client-care units, which house the clients, are central. They are usually specialized in that care is rendered to clients with similar problems, for example, medical, surgical, obstetrical, or pediatric. Other departments provide administrative, technical, diagnostic, and other types of support.

5. Hospital restructuring has included rationalizing services, discharging clients earlier, and replacing acute care with chronic care and "step-down" beds.

6. As clinical secretary, you will have clerical responsibilities (such as maintaining charts and schedules, ordering supplies, and transcribing orders) and communication responsibilities (such as answering the telephone and keeping co-workers informed). You will coordinate the unit's administrative functions and liaise with other departments. Never disregard the boundaries that define your scope of practice. If a client needs care, find a nurse.

7. In terms of choosing the work area best suited to you, try to find the department that suits your skills and personality. If you like a fast pace and cope well under pressure, you may be happy working in the Emergency Department; if you find that too stressful but enjoy detail, you may prefer the Medical Records Department.

8. Hospitals are becoming increasingly computerized, although some hospitals still keep charts and orders manually. You can become the computer expert for your unit.

9. Keep health information confidential. Never allow an unauthorized person access to client charts. Never reveal information on the telephone or in person without authorization.

10. Become familiar with your facility's security policies and emergency procedures. Learn the universal codes (or those used in your facility). Do not hesitate to ask for identification if someone you do not know is seeking access to a closed area or to client records. Most hospitals require photo ID tags. Some units are "secure" and require that visitors and staff identify themselves before entering.

Key Terms

ACUTE CARE 372	DRESSING TRAY 391	SHIFT REPORT 392
CHRONIC CARE 372	EMESIS BASIN (KIDNEY BASIN,	SPHYGMOMANOMETER 389
CLINICAL SECRETARY	K-BASIN) 378	STETHOSCOPE 389
(WARD CLERK) 386	ENDOSCOPY 381	SUBACUTE, TRANSITIONAL, OR
COLLABORATIVE PARTNERSHIP 374	LAPAROSCOPE 375	STEP-DOWN CARE 375
CREDENTIALLING 383	OPHTHALMOSCOPE 390	SUBDURAL HEMATOMA 380
CRITICALLY ILL 381	OTOSCOPE 390	SUTURE REMOVAL TRAY 391
CROSS-COVERAGE 388	PALLIATIVE CARE 379	TERMINAL CLEANING 378
DAY SURGERY 375	RATIONALIZATION OF SERVICES 375	ULTRASONOGRAPHER 382

Review Questions

1. Differentiate between an acute care or general hospital and a nursing home.

2. What is meant by a partnership agreement among hospitals?

3. What are the implications of hospital restructuring in Canada for health office professionals?

4. List the clerical and communication duties of the clinical secretary.

5. What is meant by the phrase *scope of practice?*

6. List the various parts of the client-care unit and their functions.

7. What are a clinical secretary's responsibilities in regard to equipment often kept at the nurses' station?

8. Identify three actions you could take to keep electronic charts confidential.

9. What would you do if a client threatened to leave the hospital without permission?

10. What would you do if a client had a cardiac arrest?

Application Exercises

1. Using the Internet, research the job description of the registered nurse, the registered practical nurse, and the personal support worker. List specific activities that each is qualified to carry out. Interview a family member or friend and ask him what he thinks these professionals do. Interview someone in one of these professions. Compare their answers with those other students collected and with the Internet job descriptions.

2. Interview a clinical secretary (or ward clerk). Ask her to describe her responsibilities. Compare them with those discussed in this chapter.

3. Research the organizational structure of a local hospital and what services it offers the community.

4. With another student, create a set of guidelines for maintaining confidentiality of electronic medical information on a client-care unit. Draw on research from your school or municipal library and/or the Internet.

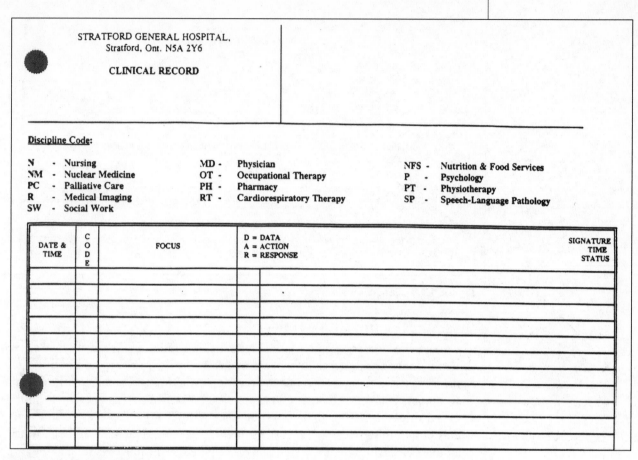

Figure 15.7   Clinical record.

Provided courtesy of Stratford General Hospital.

what the nurse is entering (e.g., Mr. Purves is complaining of incisional pain). Action is the action the nurse took to address the problem (e.g., Mr. Purves was given Demerol 100 mg IM). Response is how the client responded to the action and may be charted when a later assessment is made (e.g., Mr. Purves appears much more comfortable and stated his pain was 3 on a scale of 1 to 10). SOAP charting is another commonly used format. S stands for subjective assessments or what the client says ("I am having terrible pain"). O is for objective assessments or what the examiner sees (The client is guarding his right side and moving slowly"). A is the assessment ("The client has not had Demerol for 4 hours, his pain is incisional in nature and a stated 9 on a scale of 1 to 10"). P is for plan, what the person assessing the client—in this case the nurse—plans to do about the problem (e.g., the client was given 100 mg of Demerol IM).

In a computerized facility, these entries would be made at the computer in the nursing station or on handheld computers. They are then transferred, like all such records, to the appropriate screen in the client's computerized chart.

Progress Notes

Figure 15.8 is an example of hospital progress notes. Progress notes are used primarily by physicians and reflect the physician's assessment of the client's response to treatment while in hospital. A physician usually records progress notes each time she sees the client. There may be more than one physician who records in these notes. Each entry must be dated and signed. In a computerized environment, doctors can add notes electronically from any computer linked to the hospital system.

Conestoga General Hospital

Client   Doe John D
Hospital #   23432933
Room #   304-2
DOB   680405

January 8/04
1200 shortness of breath. 02 sats 92%. Dr. Jones notified. 02 @ 3 1 started per n/p.
resps 26, p. 100

January 9/04
0700-1900 02 ctd. Vital signs within normal range. Physio as ordered. Some crackles noted
in LLL.

January 10/04
1000 To University hospital by ambulance for MRI.

Figure 15.8 Progress notes.

Graphic Record/Vital Signs

The graphic record (see Figure 15.9) is a graphic illustration of the client's vital signs, sometimes along with other information, such as bowel movements. Routine vital signs are taken at various intervals depending on the hospital's policies, the client's condition, and the doctor's orders. Signs are usually taken at least once every 24 hours, if not once per shift, although in some long-term care facilities, they may be done only weekly or monthly. In an ICU, vital signs might be taken several times an hour. In the computerized environment, the vital signs are entered by the nurses as soon as they are taken and transferred to the electronic vital signs assessment sheet. If a client is unstable and vital signs are taken frequently, a paper recording may be used as well to allow nurses and doctors to get the information at a glance.

Medication Administration Record (MAR)

There are several sheets used to record medications. *Any* medication given to a client must be recorded and signed for. If your facility uses paper doctor's orders and MARs, keep completed MAR sheets in the chart along with doctor's orders. Keep current ones in a separate medication administration binder, which contains MARs for all clients on the unit.

A separate form is usually used for *standing* or *routine medications*—those given to a client regularly. There are also specific sheets to record *single-dose medications, patient-controlled analgesia* (discussed in Chapter 17), and *PRN* medications—those given only when needed. Most facilities also have a special medication sheet for intravenous solutions or record them electronically only (discussed in detail in Chapter 17). Hypoglycemics and anticoagulants may also be recorded on separate MARs, each allowing for the recording of related lab results (blood sugar for the hypoglycemics, APTT and INR for anticoagulants).

Signature Sheet

Some facilities keep a signature sheet in each client's chart. The purpose of this sheet is to provide a method of tracking initials. The first time a person makes entries in the chart, she must note the date, print her full name, sign her name, and provide a sample of her initials. Thereafter, her initials will serve as signature and identification.

Consultation and Laboratory Reports

A specialist who sees a client for a consultation dictates his findings. The report is sent up by Medical Records when completed, and you add it to the chart.

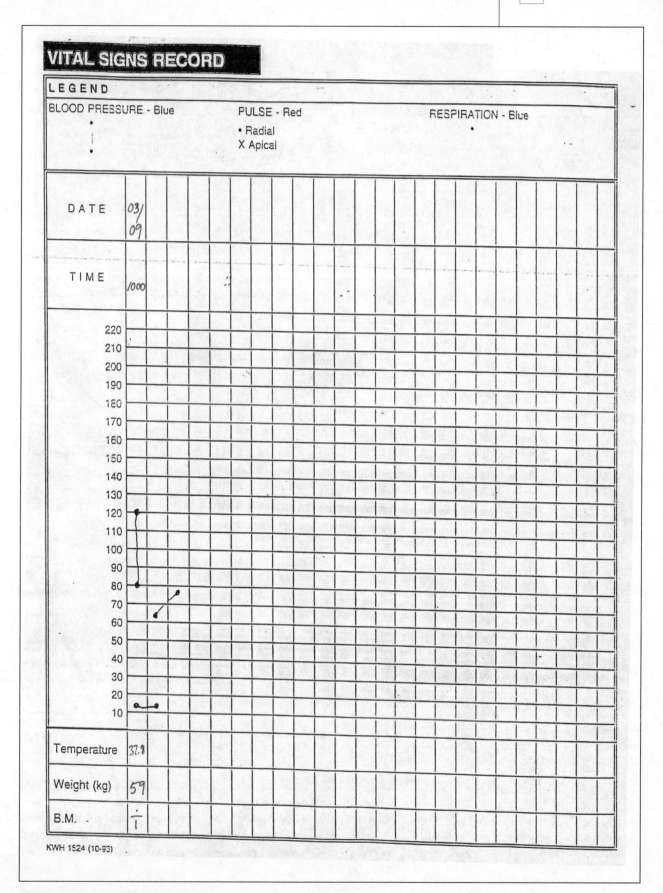

Figure 15.9   Graphic record.

Provided courtesy of Stratford General Hospital.

GENERAL HOSPITAL
MEDICATION RECORD—SCHEDULED
Check here if more than one page in use ____
See also: Diabetic Protocol ____

SCHEDULED MEDICATIONS

YEAR: _____

MONTH: _____

Start/Re-Order Date	Stop Date	Medication, Name, Dose, Route, Freq.	Hour Due						

Figure 15.10   Medication administration record.

Reports on diagnostic tests (such as X-rays, bone scans, and mammograms) are usually dictated by the physician who interprets the results and typed by a medical transcriptionist. They may be sent on paper or electronically. Ensure that electronic reports are with the appropriate file or download one for the chart. Medical Records will send a copy to the doctor who ordered the test and (if it is a different doctor) to the family doctor.

Laboratory reports (discussed extensively in Chapter 6) are usually generated by the department in the lab that processed the test, but each lab handles reports differently. The results of all lab tests, including pathology reports from surgery and biopsies, will come to the floor when they are completed. They may be sent electronically (see Figure 15.11) or in paper format. In most facilities, paper lab reports are couriered to the floor toward the end of the day shift or early in the evening shift. Add them to the charts as promptly as possible so that they are available to physicians; this also prevents the reports from being misplaced. If you use paper charts, file a hard copy in the client's chart, even if the report arrives electronically. In a computerized environment, reports are automatically attached to the electronic chart. However, you need to check to see that results of lab tests are back.

If the client has a **critical value**, usually the lab will call the doctor or the floor. If you receive a call about an abnormal value, notify the physician or the nurse immediately.

Chart Forms for Special Circumstances

A number of other forms may be added to a client's chart for special circumstances. Examples include a respiratory therapy record or a special assessment sheet for clients receiving blood. Clients who have had head injuries or surgery will be placed on **head injury routine**—a special set of checks for neurological functioning, including level of consciousness, pupil dilation, limb movement, ability to open eyes, motor response, and verbal response. These checks produce a rating on the Glasgow Coma Scale, a widely accepted means of monitoring changes in the level of consciousness. Results will be recorded on a special neurological observation record form. Clients on intravenous for

CRITICAL VALUE   a test result that so deviates from normal that it causes concern for the client's immediate well-being.

HEAD INJURY ROUTINE a special assessment for a client who has had head trauma or surgery, including checks on neurological functioning such as verbal response and pupil dilation.

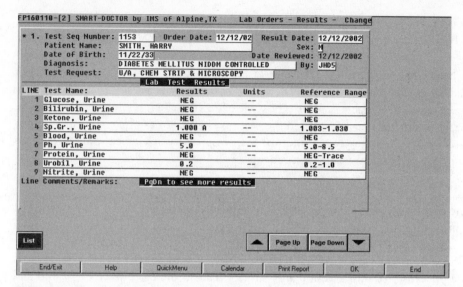

Figure 15.11 Electronic lab report (urinalysis).

Courtesy of SmartDoctor® Systems by Intelligent Medical Systems, Inc., Alpine, TX.

any reason would have an intake-and-output sheet, otherwise known as the fluid balance sheet (described under The Surgical Chart).

The Surgical Chart

A surgical chart usually starts off with the same forms as a medical chart. If a client is admitted for investigation, no additional forms may be needed. If a surgeon decides to operate, you add surgical forms to that chart. Basic surgical forms include the following:

- Consent form
- Pre-operative (pre-anesthetic) questionnaire
- History and physical assessment
- Pre-operative check list
- Anesthesia record
- Fluid balance sheet (needed for IV, which almost all OR clients have, even if briefly)
- Surgical sheets (These may include the OR instrument/sponge count checklist and the doctor's standard postoperative order sheet, if applicable. Make sure the chart contains a blank doctor's orders sheet.)

Other forms may be needed depending on the facility, the diagnosis, and the type of surgery. For example:

- Neurological postoperative assessment sheet for neurosurgery
- ECG report
- Certain lab reports (e.g., CBC, blood transfusion information)
- History and physical report if not in the chart

Pre-operative, or Pre-anesthetic Questionnaire

The client should always fill out and sign this questionnaire before any operation or procedure involving anesthetic. It typically questions clients about factors that may affect the safety of anesthetic use, including heart, lung, and kidney disease, blood pressure, diabetes, fluid retention, use of tobacco and alcohol, prior experience with anesthetics, allergies, and current medications. The nurse fills out readings of vital signs.

Clients must take with them forms regarding their treatment and medications. Fill out basic information, such as the client's name, and give the forms to the nurses to complete. You may also need to fill out a form for the ambulance. Keep a list of what documents are required.

Nutritional Services

In a computerized environment, as soon as the client's discharge order is processed, Nutritional Services receives notification of the discharge and will automatically cancel the client's dietary orders. Otherwise, call Nutritional Services with a list of discharges for the day.

Physical Resources/Housekeeping

Housekeeping needs to clean the room or bed of a discharged client to make it ready for the next client. Housekeeping may be notified electronically of discharges, but most client-care units also keep a list of discharges for their reference, often on the counter of the nurses' station. To help housekeeping plan their day's work, keep this list up-to-date, listing all planned discharges and then noting the actual times the clients leave. All rooms must be **terminally cleaned** prior to a new admission.

TERMINAL CLEANING the bed and other furniture used by the client are thoroughly cleaned with a specifically selected disinfectant solution.

Disassembling the Chart

When a client is discharged, remove the components of the chart from the binder, and place them in a specific order according to hospital protocol. In most hospitals, remove the MAR from the medication binder and add it to the disassembled chart. Check that the nurses have completed and signed a discharge summary and initialed all medications they have given on the MAR. Make sure the time of discharge has been added to the face sheet. When the client has left and all charting is completed, send the chart to Medical Records. Electronic charts are also filed or stored in Medical Records, and you must do a similar check for completeness. There is a space on the face sheet usually marked LOS, for length of stay. You would enter the number of hospital days in that area or field. The client's discharge diagnosis and any surgical procedures are also listed on the face sheet. Often, the doctor will fill these areas in when he signs the discharge order. If you are not allowed to do this, ask the nurses to complete it. The information is usually on the client's progress notes.

Unauthorized Departures

If a client insists on leaving the hospital without a physician's order, ask her to sign a release form stating that she is leaving without permission, therefore assuming responsibility for her own health. However, a client who insists on leaving is often upset or angry and may refuse to sign the form. Ask a nurse to deal with the situation. Until the nurse arrives, be polite, and try to keep the client calm. Notify the doctor as soon as possible. The nurses will make the appropriate documentation on the client's chart. If the client leaves before the nurse arrives, you may be asked to chart what occurred. Be clear and concise. Quote directly what you can remember of the conversation. For example:

Mr. Barrera said, "I am leaving. This place has caused me nothing but trouble." He turned and left.

Stick to the facts. Do not give your impressions or make assumptions. For example, instead of writing "He was angry and upset," write "He appeared to be angry and upset."

Deaths

When a client dies, a doctor—or sometimes a nurse—confirms that the client is deceased. A death certificate must be filled out and signed by a doctor. Then, you can call the morgue once the body can be released from the floor. In smaller facilities that do not always have a doctor around, the nurse will call a doctor when a death occurs. Occasionally, when a death has been expected and occurs in the middle of the night, the doctor may authorize a nurse to release the body and will sign the death certificate when he arrives at the hospital in the morning. This will also be subject to the wishes of the family. Sometimes religious and/or cultural beliefs or practices determine when the body can be moved. Disassemble the chart in the usual manner.

In some provinces, the coroner reviews randomly selected hospital deaths. The family may be required to pay a fee, even though they did not request a coroner's review. Requests for organ donation, when appropriate, are handled by the doctor or the nurses.

If you think grieving family members need privacy, direct them to the hospital chapel, if you have one, or to an empty conference or meeting room.

Transfers

Sometimes, clients are transferred from one unit to another within the hospital, usually on a doctor's order, either for medical reasons, such as to receive surgery that the original unit cannot offer, or to provide appropriate accommodation. Remove the chart from the client's binder, but do not disassemble it, and send it with the client to the new unit. Make sure all the client's belongings, medications, hospital card, and MARs go with him.

Other Standard Files and Resources

As well as the forms used in the charts, you will be filing or keeping on hand a number of forms, resources, and teaching materials. Each client-care unit (even if computerized) keeps a supply of blank forms such as permission/consent forms, release-of-responsibility forms, and history forms.

Requisitions

A requisition is simply an order form. Chapter 6 discussed requisitions for diagnostic tests. These are required for most laboratory and diagnostic tests in hospital; however, requisitions are also needed for such services as a dietary consultation. A requisition must contain the client's identifying information (hard copies are addressographed), the details of the request, and any other relevant information. You fill in the latter when transcribing the doctor's orders (discussed in the next chapter).

In a computerized environment, requisitions are electronic. For example, you would send a request for a CBC to the lab electronically, where it would be filed in their system until processed. The lab would print out a label for the specimen and send a report electronically. Whether the requisition is paper or electronic, if an appointment is required, the clinical secretary in the lab would book it and notify the client-care unit.

Orders for specimens collected by nurses (such as urine, sputum, or stool) also require requisitions. In computerized facilities, they may be computer generated and printed right in the nursing unit.

Paper-based requisitions are often in duplicate, and a copy is kept in the chart. When ordering a test or service electronically, some systems automatically note the order and the date results are expected in the lab section of the PI screen.

Community Agency Forms

For many clients, discharge planning involves support from a community agency. Agencies require referral and assessment forms before setting up support. In a paper system, file the blank forms alphabetically by agency. In a computerized environment, the forms are available online.

Teaching Material

Many client-care units keep preprinted health teaching information of various types. These may be given to the client during the hospital stay or upon discharge. An example of this would be postoperative self-care following a hip replacement or physiotherapy instructions.

TPR Book

Units that are not computerized record clients' vital signs (temperature, pulse, and respirations, or TPR) and bowel movements in a book. It is your responsibility to prepare and update this book daily. Each day's section contains a list of all clients in the unit, with headers indicating the times at which vital signs are recorded. Most units take vital signs routinely o.d. (daily) or b.i.d. Clients with an elevated temperature, pulse, or respiration rate may have them taken more often. Blood pressures are not usually recorded in this book.

Lab Book

Some clinical secretaries keep a book to record lab results that are telephoned or faxed in. Keeping all records in one place makes them easy to refer to and prevents loss of bits of loose paper. The information must be complete: client's full name, hospital number, room number, bed number, doctor, and the lab results. Also record the name of the person from whom you took the results. Remember to read back the results for accuracy. Initial or sign any results you record.

Daily Assignment Schedule

You may be responsible for keeping a list of the clients in the unit. The charge nurse or clinical leader will use this to assign staff. Once she has added the names of the nurses looking after particular clients, it becomes a staff assignment sheet, as shown in Figure 15.15. It may also designate break and lunch times.

List of Admissions and Discharges

In some facilities, the clinical secretary will post a list of all known admissions and discharges, adding to it as changes occur. Nurses will incorporate this information into their daily schedule so they know whom to prepare for discharge and know how many admissions to expect. In other units, this information is written on the side of the assignment schedule.

Rho(d) immunoglobulin (WinRho) is added to standard orders and applies to RH-negative mothers. An RH-negative mother who has an RH-positive baby must receive this medication within 72 hours of delivery to prevent the formation of antibodies that could pose risk to a subsequent baby if that baby is RH positive.

MMR refers to the measles-mumps-rubella vaccine. If the mother's blood test shows that she is not immune to rubella, usually vaccination is given before she leaves the hospital to prevent exposing any future fetuses to the rubella virus, which can be teratogenic (harmful) in the first trimester of pregnancy.

STANDARD PRE-ADMISSION ORDERS Pre-admission orders are those completed prior to the client's admission to hospital. This applies to clients who come in for procedures and are discharged the same day (Day Surgery) and to clients admitted the morning of their surgery but who will be staying one night or more (Admit Same Day or ASD clients), and for those who are admitted the night (or more) before a procedure. Other necessary pre-operative pre-parations (unless the client is an in-patient) are carried out at home. These may include an enema or a laxative, and remaining NPO after a certain time, usually 2200hrs. This is important because an anesthetic may cause the client to vomit any food in the stomach. Vomit could accidentally be aspirated (taken into the lungs), which might cause problems, including a respiratory arrest.

As you can see in Figure 16.5, these orders include blood work that is ordered by a code system. Code A shows that only a complete blood count (CBC) needs to be done, and so on. Major surgery requires more blood work (including preparations in case the client needs a blood transfusion), an electrocardiogram, and a chest X-ray. Many facilities routinely do ECGs on clients over a certain age, usually over 40 or 50 years. Note also that on this sheet, there are orders related to the client's discharge. There is a saying that the client's discharge begins on admission, which certainly is reflected here.

Electronic Doctor's Orders

Some hospitals use electronic doctor's orders, as shown in Figure 16.6. The physician enters the orders directly into the computer, using a password and a specialized computer-based signature.

Requisitions

In a noncomputerized environment, you will want to have requisition forms handy while transcribing orders (see Chapters 6 and 15). Requisitions are seldom, if ever, used in the computerized environment. Instead, you would select the appropriate laboratory department, enter the type of test, the date and time the test is to be done, the urgency, who will obtain the test, and any necessary clinical information. File or send the request, which will be received electronically in the appropriate department.

The Client Care Activity Record

Many orders are recorded on a main client care summary, or health record. In a manual environment, that document is often called a **kardex** (the most common proprietary name). If all orders are transcribed electronically, they will be recorded on an electronic client care summary record, or electronic health record, also called a **patient intervention screen (PI screen)** or patient activity screen. Many facilities informally call the electronic client care summary record an "electronic kardex" because it fulfills the same function. The kardex or PI screen is a centralized source of information that begins with admission and addresses almost every component of the client's diagnosis, treatment, and care while in the hospital. Nurses may print it out and carry it as a guide. Throughout the following chapters, I will refer to the kardex or PI

KARDEX commonly used proprietary name for a paper-based client care document or health record.

PATIENT INTERVENTION SCREEN (PI SCREEN) or **ELECTRONIC HEALTH RECORD** a computer-based client care document containing the same information as a kardex. This is an electronic version of a traditional kardex.

Duplicate Doctor's Order Form
Detach Part 2 and Send to Pharmacy

STRATFORD GENERAL HOSPITAL

☐ DAY SURGERY
☐ DAY SURGERY - SHORT STAY
☐ ASD
☐ INPATIENT

PRE-ADMISSION ORDERS

Detach Part 2 and Send to Pharmacy

OBTAIN CONSENT FOR _____
(Name of OR Procedure)

LABORATORY TESTS:

☐ CODE A – CBC

☐ CODE B – CBC, Diff, BUN
    Creatinine Electrolytes
    Random Glucose

☐ PT   PTT

☐ Electrolytes (for all Patients On Diuretics)

☐ CODE U – CBC & Diff, BUN,
    Creatinine Electrolytes,
    Random Glucose, Urinalysis,
    Urine Culture & Sensitivity

☐ CODE Z – No Bloodwork Required

☐ HCG (required for all Gyn patients under 50)

☐ Urine Culture & Sensitivity

☐ Group & Reserve Serum

☐ Cross Match & Type for _____ Units

☐ ECG (Required for all patients age 40 & over)

Other Laboratory

Tests _____

_____

PRE-OPERATIVE CONSULTATION REQUESTED

☐ Cardiorespiratory Services

☐ ABG   ☐ Oximetry   ☐ Spirometry

☐ CBG

☐ Abbreviated Pulmonary Function Tests

☐ Other _____

☐ Home Care

Specify _____

_____

☐ Anaesthesiologist Consultation

☐ Social Services

Specify _____

_____

☐ Other _____

_____

DIAGNOSTIC IMAGING

☐ Chest X-Ray

Other _____

Other Orders: _____

_____

FOR HOSPITAL USE ONLY

OR Booking _____
               (Date & Time)

Clinic Appointment _____
               (Date & Time)

Date _____   Physician's Signature _____
     YY MM DD
DR-036 1994/03

Figure 16.5 Standard pre-admission orders.

Provided courtesy Stratford General Hospital.

Bell, James R
234 Isobel Street
Regina, Saskatchewan
R34 7N4
Hospital no. 12343333
Room 432-2

Gravol 50 mg IM or po q3-4h prn
Demerol 75-100 mg IM q 4h prn for pain
Digoxin 0.25 mg po qam
Lasix 40 mg po qam.

January 22/04 2200hrs

Dr. Martin Price.
end of order--

Figure 16.6   Electronic doctor's orders.

screen. Keep in mind that your facility may call this summary document by a different name. Many examples in this Part of the textbook are illustrated with a kardex-type form. You will quite likely be using some electronic equivalent; the important thing to note is the information captured. Just what is added to the kardex or PI screen depends on facility guidelines.

The precise format of the kardex in any facility will vary. Often, different units within the same hospital will have variations tailored to meet the unit's need. A post-partum kardex, for example, contains, in addition to such standard items as diet and medication, information related to breastfeeding and mother–baby interaction, while a surgical kardex reports assessment of the client's incision, pain control, and fluid intake. Some facilities use a set of preprinted sheets organized according to room number and kept in a binder. Other facilities keep sheets in a rectangular plastic or metal holder filled with graduated plastic inserts, one for each room and bed number (see Figure 16.7). This is the format adopted for use in this text. You will notice that there are variations in the kardex examples used in the following chapters. Most client-care units have two or three kardexes, each containing information on a designated number of clients (often divided into groups for the puspose of assigning RNs and RPNs (nursing teams) to care for them. PI screens contain the same information as the kardex; the exact appearance of the screen differs with each software system.

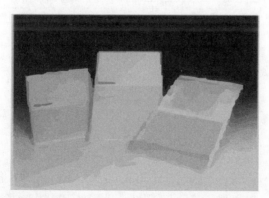

Figure 16.7   Kardex holder.

Figure 16.8 (a and b) shows an example of a kardex. The rest of this section expands on the categories shown in this figure.

Star/.order date	DAILY MEDICATIONS Medicine requiring hold/special orders	Disc Date	Start/or der date	PRN MEDICATIONS	Disc Date
				INTRAVENOUS ORDERS	
	SUPPORT IN HOSPITAL			Primary	
	Social Worker				
	Physiotherapist			Secondary	
	Dietitian				
	Vision/Hearing/Dentures			Change tubing/restart q 3 days	
	Other				
				Saline/hep lock	
				Flush:	
	TRANSFER			Other:	
	DISCHARGE PLANNING			Intake/Output	
	Community Care Agency				
	Other:				
	Date notified:			RELEVANT HISTORY	
	Services Required:				
				ALLERGIES	

Client's Name_____ Id #_____

Figure 16.8a Kardex for a surgical client, top portion.

TEACHING / EMOTIONAL SUPPORT	DATE	ELIMINATION	DATE	OTHER DIRECT CARE/ASSESSMENTS	DATE	DIAGNOSTIC TESTS	Date done
Pre/op		Self/Assist		Height/weight		X-RAYS	
Post/op		BOWEL		Abdominal Assessment			
Routine		Enema		FP Blood Sugar			
Extra		Other		Urine testing			
Other/Comments		BLADDER		CSM			
ADL: Self/Assist		Catheter		Other			
Comments:		Foley		Skin care			
		Remove/insert		ROM			
		3-way		Turn/position			
		Suprabubic		Other			
		Condom					
		Other:					
VITAL SIGNS		HYGIENE		Dressing			
Q shift		Shower/tub/bedside		Type/location			
Q shift x 2		Self		Reduction			
Q shift x 3		Assist X1 / X2		Change/Assess			
Q shift x 4		Nurse		Comments:			
Post-op routine:				Clip/Suture removal			
				Other:		LAB	
		RESPIRATIRY					
ACTIVITY:		Oxygen					
AAT / BRP/ Bed rest		Mask/ Nasal prongs:		PROCEDURES			
Self/Assist		Litres:		INSERTION/REMOVAL OF			
Other:		Oximetry		TUBES AND DRAINS			
RESTRAINTS:		Inhalation Rx		NG tube			
Type:		Spirometer		Gomco: Suction:			
Comments:		Chest Physio		Sump drain			
		Chest Assessments		Wound drain			
DIET:		Other		Hemovac			
Self/Assist:		Suctioning		Other:			
Type							
NPO				Level of Care Directives:			
Tube Feeds							
				ADVANCED/CONSTANT CARE:			
SURGERY							
DIAGNOSIS							
ADM DATE							

Room_____ Name_____ Id #_____
Doctor_____

Figure 16.8b Kardex for a surgical client, bottom portion.

Medications

Some facilities keep a current record of all medications on the client's kardex or electronic chart (as shown here). Many facilities, however, record medications (other than intravenous) only on the MAR.

		Black, Roger
	CBC	123 Duncan St.
	Electrolytes	Stratford ON N5A 2G3
	Urine for C&S	M 22 09 47 071608
K/MS	Valium 5 mg po hs prn	3238494232
K/MS	Lasix 20 mg od p o	Hanson, G. Dr.
K/MS	Demerol 75 mg IM stat noted	
K/MS	HCT 12.5 mg od p o	
K/MS	Enalapril 5 mg BID p o	
K/MS	Eltroxin 0.1 mg od p o	
K/MS	Demerol 50-100 mg q4h prn IM	
K/MS	Gravol 50 mg q4h prn IM	

date	time	Physician's printed name	Signature
Jan 2/04	1000	Dr. G. Hanson	*Dr. G Hanson*

Figure 16.11   The same doctor's orders for Mr. Black, with medications highlighted and tracking codes added after all the medications have been processed.

Black, Roger
123 Duncan St.
Stratford ON N5A 2G3

M 22 09 47 071608

3238494232

Hanson, G. Dr.

SINGLE DOSE MEDICATIONS (note: single dose and PRN orders are on one med sheet

DATE	MEDICATION, DOSE, ROUTE	TIME	INITIALS
JAN 02/04	*DEMEROL 100 MG. IM STAT*	*0100*	(nurse giving med)

PRN Medications

Start/ Re-Order	Stop date	Med, Name, Dose, Route Frequency	Jan 2			Jan 3			Jan 4			Jan 5			Jan 6		
			T	D	I	T	D	I	T	D	I	T	D	I	T	D	I
Jan 2		Valium 5 mg po hs prn															
Jan 2	Jan 5	Demerol 50-75 mg IM qh prn															
Jan 2 @1000	Jan 5 @1000	Gravol 50 mg IM q4h prn															

Figure 16.12   Single-dose and PRN MAR sheet.

◆ Mary writes "MS" on the order form beside Demerol, meaning transcribed to the med sheet, and "noted," meaning that she has notified the nurse about the stat order.

The nurse takes the MAR record, prepares the medication, gives Mr. Black the Demerol, initials the MAR, and puts it back in the binder or gives it back to Mary. In some hospitals, as further verification, a nurse who gives a stat medication also initials or signs the doctor's written order for the medication, along with the date and the word "given."

Step 3: Completing the Medication Orders

Having completed the stat order, Mary decides to finish processing the medication orders, then the lab orders, then the client care and activity orders. She has already stamped the PRN MAR and entered the single dose for the Demerol appropriately. She will use the PRN MAR sheet for the other PRN orders. Now she identifies the scheduled MAR sheet (see Figure 16.13) and stamps it with Mr. Black's information using his hospital card and the addressograph. She sits down at her desk, beside the computer and the telephone.

Processing Scheduled Medications

◆ Mary carefully copies the medications onto Mr. Black's MAR. She includes the date on which the medication is started.

◆ She enters the dose, route, and frequency, making very sure to enter numbers accurately.

◆ On the basis of the frequency ordered, Mary works out the times when medications should be given, according to facility policy, and enters those times.

◆ The scheduled medications include Enalapril, Lasix, HCT (hydrochlorothiazide), and Eltroxin. As she transcribes each medication, Mary writes the transcription code beside it. In this example, Mary uses K, meaning she has copied the medication to the kardex, and MS, meaning she has also copied it to the MAR.

◆ Mary checks that she has included all the necessary information for each medication. She leaves the stop date blank because the order did not give a stop date (these medications are required for the duration of the hospital stay). (See Table 16.1 for a detailed explanation of the components of the MAR.)

Table 16.1 | Components of Transcribed Medication Orders

(as shown in Figures 16.12 and 16.13)

Name	The name of the drug as the physician ordered it
Dose	The amount of the drug the patient is to receive (e.g., Lasix 20 mg)
Frequency	How often the medication is to be given (e.g., Lasix od or daily)
Route	How the medication is to be given. Mostly ordered po here. Demerol and Gravol were ordered IM.
Times	Based on ordered frequency. Usually, it is best to space the medication as evenly as possible (see Chapter 7).
Start Order	The start date (shown in the first column in Figure 16.13) is the date on which the order should be implemented. If the doctor does not specify otherwise, the start date is the same as the date on which the order was written (Jan. 2, in this case).
Stop Date	The stop date (second column in Figure 16.13) is not always filled out. All controlled drugs have automatic stop dates. The more common ones, such as Demerol and morphine, will have automatic stop dates ranging from 48 to 72 hours.
	Antibiotics often have automatic stop dates of seven days unless otherwise stated. Most facilities review all medications each month. Clients rarely stay that long in an acute care hospital, but long-term-care or nursing facilities often use a standard one-month stop date.

Black, Roger
123 Duncan St.
Stratford ON N5A 2G3
M 22 09 47   071608
3238494232
Hanson, D. Dr.

Start/reorder	Stop date	Medication, dose, route, frequency	Hour Due	Jan 2	Jan 3	Jan 4	Jan 5	Jan 6	Jan 7	Jan 8
Jan 02/04		Lasix, 20 mg OD p.o.	0800							
Jan 02/04		Eltroxin 0.1 mg p.o.	1000							
Jan 02/04		HCT 12.5 mg od p.o.	1000							
Jan 02/04		Enalapril 5 mg Bid p.o.	1000							
			1800							

Figure 16.13   Scheduled MAR.

Processing PRN Medication Orders

Next, Mary is going to transcribe her PRN medication orders. These include Demerol, Valium, and Gravol. She goes back to the PRN medication sheet (see Figure 16.12), on which she has already entered the stat order. Now, Mary carefully transcribes each PRN medication from the doctor's order sheet to this PRN record, making sure to copy exactly what the doctor wrote, including the medication, dose, route, and frequency.

Note that all narcotic analgesics have automatic stop dates unless otherwise specified by the doctor. Mary's hospital uses a stop date of 72 hours for Demerol, so Mary counts forward three days from the start date and puts a stop date of January 5. If a client still needs the drug after the stop date, the nurses will ask the clinical secretary to ask the doctor for a renewal or reorder. In a noncomputerized environment, you could leave a note on the client's chart or call the doctor. In a computerized environment, there is usually a "bulletin board" or "message board" somewhere in the client's electronic chart where you would write the request. The physician should check this message board regularly.

In the columns under the dates in Figure 16.12,

◆ T means the time the medication was given,

◆ D is for dose, meaning the dose given, and

◆ I is for the nurse's initials.

On a MAR with this format, you must remember to leave enough lines for the nurses to initial each time they give the medication. If the Demerol is ordered q4h, that means that, in 24 hours, the client could have a maximum of six doses (24 divided by 4). Therefore, Mary needs to leave at least six lines.

Dose Range for PRN Medications

Some PRN medication orders are written with a dose range. In this case, the doctor ordered a range of 50–75 mg of Demerol, meaning the nurse may give the client either 50 or 75 mg, depending on how bad the client's pain is. The nurse may make this decision in consultation with the client. A pain scale is a helpful assessment tool. The client is asked to assign a number between 1 and 5 (or 1 and 10) to the pain he is currently experiencing, with 0 as no pain and 5 (or 10) as the worst pain he has ever experienced.

Frequencies for PRN medications are maximums and provide safety parameters. Q4h means that the medication may be given no more often than every four hours. Some doctors order a range, such as q3–4 hrs. The Demerol, for example, could be given every three hours if needed. Often, nurses will give it as much as a half-hour earlier, but no sooner. This is considered appropriate by most facilities.

These orders are now complete. Mary rechecks her orders, has the nurse check her orders, and signs off. She tears off the back copy and sends it to Pharmacy. She returns the chart to the appropriate place.

Discontinuing Existing Orders

Only a physician may discontinue an order. Occasionally, a doctor will order a medication discontinued at a specific time, for example, d/c after 1800. Otherwise, the medication should be discontinued as soon as the order is received. The clinical secretary or nurse must go to the appropriate MAR record and write d/c in the appropriate spot after the last dose to be given or that has been given. It is a good idea to shade the area after the last dose to be given. For example, Dr. Hanson comes in on January 3. He decides that Mr. Black no longer needs HCT as a diuretic (he is also on Lasix, a diuretic sometimes used in combination with HCT). He also finds that Mr. Black has become increasingly anxious and feels that prescribing Valium throughout the day as well as at night may help. Mary finds Mr. Black's chart on her desk, flagged to notify her that there was a new order (Figure 16.14).

- Mary checks the order (Figure 16.14) to be sure it is stamped with Mr. Black's addressograph information. She ensures the order is dated and signed by Dr. Hanson. She checks for allergies on the order sheet.
- Next, Mary again scans the order for anything urgent or stat, noting that there are only two medication orders.
- The medication orders must be transcribed to Mr. Black's medication administration records, so she gets them out of the medication binder, which is on the medication cart. She needs both the PRN and the scheduled MAR.
- The first order is to discontinue or stop Mr. Black's HCT. To do this, Mary clearly marks d/c on the MAR record so that the nurses do not give it when it is due next. This would be 1000 on January 4, as it has already been given for January 3. (See the HCT order in Figure 16.15.)
- Mary adds the Valium order to the scheduled medication sheet. To make it clear that Valium is to start on January 3, Mary puts diagonal lines through the signature boxes on January 2 to avoid any misreading and clearly notes the start time to avoid the possibility of confusion.
- Mary verbally notifies the nurses of the changes.

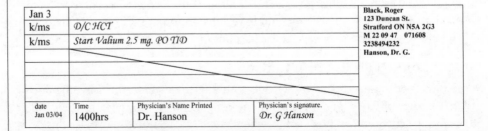

Figure 16.14   Doctor's order sheet showing new orders.

Key Terms

BOLUS 459	KARDEX 443	PATIENT INTERVENTION SCREEN
DOCTORS' ORDERS 436	LOADING DOSE 459	(PI SCREEN) 443
EPISIOTOMY 442	ORDER TRANSCRIPTION (ORDER	POSTPARTUM 442
FLAG 450	ENTRY, ORDER DISPENSATION,	PROPHYLACTIC 462
HEMOVAC 449	ORDER PROCESSING) 436	

Review Questions

1. What are the basic tools necessary to begin transcribing doctor's orders?

2. Where does the process of order transcription begin?

3. What elements must be present on the doctor's order sheet before you can begin transcribing the orders?

4. What are standard doctor's orders, and when are they used?

5. Summarize the information recorded in a kardex or a PI screen.

6. Why are physicians asked to flag charts? What are the clinical secretary's related responsibilities?

7. What must you do when you have finished transcribing a client's orders?

8. Differentiate between routine or standing medication orders, PRN, stat, and sliding-scale medication orders.

9. When might a medication ticket be used?

10. Why is it important for you to add a client's medication administration records to the client's preoperative chart?

Application Exercises

1. Research a hospital or other health-care facility near you. Interview a clinical secretary or someone in the Medical Records Department. Find out what kind of doctor's order forms, medication administration records, and kardex or health records are used. How many paper forms are used, and how many records are electronic? In what ways do the forms differ from those shown in this chapter? Are there any specific policies about transcription that are not described in this chapter?

2. Using the MAR format used by a local hospital, or one supplied by your instructor, transcribe the following orders written by Dr. Smith for Alison Chambers.

   Demerol 75–100 mg IM q3–4h PRN
   Gravol 50 mg IM or PO q4 h PRN for nausea
   Magnolax 30 cc bid start day 3 PRN
   Tylenol 3 po q4h PRN

3. Using the same MAR format as in question 2, transcribe the following orders written by Dr. Martello for Alia Hondo. Alia is diabetic and has a urinary tract infection.

   Insulin Novolin 30/70 20 units qam and 7 units
     ac supper
   Insulin Novolin R 10 units stat
   Insulin by reaction Novolin R 5 units if BS greater
     than 15 qam
   Finger-prick blood sugar readings qid
   Lasix 20 mg q2days
   Septra DS I tab bid × 7 days

4. You have just received new orders for Mr. Black. Working from the medication sheet shown in Figure 16.32, transcribe the following orders:

   Increase Lasix to 40 mg od
   Start Wellbutrin 150 mg bid
   Heparin 5000 units s/c q 12 h
   Tylenol plain 325 1 tab q4h for temp above 38
   D/C Valium

Start/reorder	Stop date	Medication dose, route, frequency	Hour Due	Jan 2	Jan 3	Jan 4	Jan 5	Jan 6
Jan 02/04		Lasix, 20 mg. po od	0800					
Jan 02/04		Eltroxin 0.1 mg po od	1000					
Jan 02/04		Enalapril 5 mg po	1000					
		bid	1800					
Jan 02/04		HCT 12.5 mg po od	1000			DC		
Jan 04/04		Valium 2.5 mg po	1000		Start			
		t.i.d.	1400		↓			
			1800					

Figure 16.32   Medication sheet for Exercise 4.

CHAPTER 17

Orders for Intravenous Therapy

On completing this chapter, you will be able to:

1. Explain what homeostasis is and list the main elements responsible for fluid and electrolyte balance in the body.
2. Discuss the indications for and goals of intravenous therapy.
3. Describe the equipment involved in intravenous therapy.
4. Summarize the purpose and advantages of an electronic infusion pump.
5. Explain the advantages of patient-controlled analgesia.
6. Effectively transcribe orders related to intravenous infusion.
7. Effectively transcribe orders related to intravenous medications.
8. Discuss the indications for blood product transfusion.
9. List the more common blood products and their uses.

Intravenous (IV) therapy is a common hospital treatment and is often critical to the hospitalized client's recovery. With the current emphasis on home-based care, clients can also be discharged and maintained on parenteral therapy in the home under the supervision of community nurses. Intravenous means "into the vein," when fluids are introduced directly into the body's circulatory system. Intravenous therapy is prescribed for people requiring electrolyte replacement, fluids, calories, vitamins, or other nutritional substances. It is also a route for administering medications, including chemotherapy, and is used for transfusion of blood products.

To accurately transcribe IV orders, you need to understand the purposes and goals of IV therapy, the equipment involved, and the types of solutions ordered by physicians. This chapter will briefly discuss the more common types of intravenous solutions, intravenous medications, and blood and blood products.

Although intravenous solutions themselves are not, strictly speaking, medications, in some facilities they are treated and recorded in much the same manner because they involve introducing something external into the body system.

INTRAVENOUS (IV) administered directly into the circulatory system via a vein.

Fluids and Electrolytes

To fully understand the purpose and goals of IV therapy, you need a basic understanding of the roles that fluids and electrolytes play in maintaining the body's equilibrium.

Electrolyte is a term for salts or ions that dissolve in water and have electrical charges. Salt or sodium (Na), potassium (K), and chloride (Cl) are the three major electrolytes our bodies need to function properly. Imbalances in sodium may be caused by inappropriate fluid loss or retention. Potassium imbalances can cause

				Parenteral Therapy:	
			Jan 2	IV 1000cc 2/3 and 1/3 @ 100cc/hr. alternate with	
				1000 N/S with 20 meq KCL	
				Restart IV/change tubing	
				Q 3 days Jan 4, 5, 8, 11	
Discharge:					
				Messages:	
				Relevant past history	
SURGERY:	AGE:				
	ADMISSION DATE:			ALLERGIES	
DIAGNOSIS:	PRIMARY:				
	SECONDARY:				

Figure 17.12   Bottom portion of a kardex showing IV order.

Blood Transfusions

A physician who wants to order blood replacement for a client can choose from several blood products depending on the client's need and diagnosis and sometimes on the client's wishes. The client may refuse to have a blood transfusion for personal or religious reasons. Jehovah's Witnesses, for example, usually refuse to receive any blood or blood products because they believe the Bible prohibits them to do so. For the most part, their right to refuse treatment is respected, although there have been cases where the province has overridden the parents' wishes when a physician believes the transfusion is necessary for the child's survival.

Reasons for Blood Transfusion

Doctors most commonly order blood transfusion as prophylaxis for a client undergoing major surgery, to treat anemia, or to treat blood loss from hemorrhage. Other blood products are administered for various reasons. For example, factor VIII is given to hemophiliacs for clotting, often with other components in the form of a solution called cryoprecipitate.

Prophylaxis

Most surgeons will order blood, usually packed cells (see explanation below) to be available for clients having major surgery in case of excessive blood loss during surgery. Blood will be cross-matched for a client and held in the lab for her. If she does not need the blood, it will be released and available for another suitable recipient.

Anemia

Anemia is characterized by too few red blood cells in a person's blood. There are a number of causes for this. Severe anemia is usually treated with the infusion of packed cells.

Start/reorder	Stop date	Medication, dose, route, frequency	Hour Due	Jan 1	Jan 2	Jan 3	Jan 4	Jan 5	Jan 6	Jan 7
Jan 02/04		Ancef 1 g Q6h	0600							
		IV	1200							
			1800							
			2200							

Figure 17.13   Scheduled MAR showing antibiotic to be administered by minibag.

Acute Blood Loss

Any situation in which a person loses an excessive amount of blood (usually by definition over 750 cc) is called a hemorrhage. This causes the body to go into shock. The most effective way to treat massive hemorrhage is by blood replacement.

Preparation

Before receiving a blood transfusion, a client must be cross-matched and typed first (that is, his blood type and Rh factor among other things must be determined) to ensure that he receives compatible blood. Otherwise a serious reaction could occur. The physician will order the type of blood or blood product the client is to receive.

Types of Blood Products

Whole Blood

If a doctor orders whole blood, it will be ordered as a unit of blood: approximately 520 cc of donated blood. It may be used to treat excessive blood loss resulting from trauma, surgery, or burns. Whole blood is not frequently ordered.

Platelets

Platelets are extracted from whole blood and ordered for someone with thrombocytopenia, or a low blood platelet count. Anyone with low platelets is at risk for bleeding disorders, in particular disseminated intravascular coagulopathy (DIC), a potentially fatal condition characterized by widespread bleeding. Platelets, too, are ordered by the unit.

Fresh Frozen Plasma

Plasma, derived from whole blood, contains all coagulation, or clotting, factors and is given to clients with coagulation defects. One unit is usually approximately 225 cc.

Packed Cells

The most commonly ordered blood product is packed cells: red blood cells separated from whole blood by a process called centrifugation. Packed blood cells may be used to correct anemia when extra volume is not desirable for a client, for example, in the case of congestive heart failure. Because it does not contain white blood cells, it poses less risk of minor reactions. A doctor might order "Cross and type for two units of packed cells" or "C·T for 2 units of packed cells on cross match for two units of packed cells."

Albumin

This is a protein extracted from the blood and is often used to expand fluid volume within the blood vessels.

Cryoprecipitate

Cryoprecipitate is part of the fresh frozen plasma that contains a clotting factor called factor VIII. It is most commonly given to hemophiliacs to help control bleeding.

The Blood Transfusion Process and the Clinical Secretary's Responsibilities

While procedures vary from one hospital to another, the following section outlines the typical process. If the blood is ordered for someone who is going for major surgery, the person will be cross-matched and typed. The selection and amount of blood product ordered will be prepared for the client and held in the blood bank until used, or until it is clear that the client will not need it. The blood bank will send a list of the units prepared for the client. Each unit of blood product will be assigned an identification number. Always note it down on the kardex or PI screen if blood is being held for a client.

Whether manually or electronically, a requisition is sent to the blood bank, and the blood bank notifies the floor when the blood product is ready. If it is to be given as soon as available, someone from the client care unit will go to the lab to pick it up. You may occasionally be asked to do this. If so, you must complete a series of checks with the lab technologist to ensure that you are getting precisely what has been ordered for the client. Bring the floor's copy of the blood requisition and/or the client's addressograph card. Check this information against the unit of blood product being sent to the floor and against the ledger in which the same information is recorded. Check the blood product again with the nurses, confirming the client's name, hospital number, room number, blood type, and the number assigned to the unit of blood product.

In a manual environment, you may need to addressograph a special vital signs graph used for clients receiving transfusions. The nurses check the client's vital signs frequently to detect any reaction, especially in the first hour when reactions are most likely. In a computerized environment, the nurses would enter the vital signs electronically. Even in computerized environments, sometimes, vital signs taken frequently are documented on paper also.

Hyperalimentation or Total Parenteral Nutrition

Hyperalimentation or total parenteral nutrition (TPN) is the intravenous administration of nutrients to clients who cannot absorb food through their gastrointestinal tract. This is discussed in Chapter 18.

Summary

1. Our health depends on a balance of fluids and electrolytes, known as homeostasis. Healthy people take this balance for granted and maintain it naturally. Our bodies correct imbalances; for example, thirst prompts us to maintain fluid levels. The most common elements in maintaining homeostasis are sodium, potassium, and chloride. These electronically charged ions assist with the transport of nutrients within the body and contribute to muscle and nerve functions. Sick people are especially at risk for fluid and electrolyte imbalances.

2. Intravenous therapy is used to correct electrolyte imbalances, maintain homeostasis, deliver medications, and supply blood products, when needed. It is used to rehydrate clients or maintain hydration and fluid balance in clients who cannot eat or drink because of disease, trauma, or surgery.

3. Infusion can be started with an intracatheter, a butterfly needle, or a peripherally inserted central catheter (PICC), a more stable line into the vena cava for long-term use. Various types of tubing are available depending on the client's needs.

4. IV solutions may be delivered by gravity, with the rate controlled by roller clamps, or by various types of pumps. Patient-controlled analgesia (PCA) pumps allow clients to administer their own pain relief as needed. Small portable pumps, some of which are computer assisted (e.g., CAD), allow patients with terminal or chronic illnesses to manage pain at home.

5. A range of solutions are available; among the more common are D5W (5% dextrose in water), 2/3 and 1/3 (3.3% glucose and 0.3% sodium chloride), normal saline (0.9% NaCl in water), and Ringer's lactate, a solution of sodium, potassium, calcium, and chloride.

6. Intravenous medication is administered in three ways: directly into the vein (an IV push), mixed in the solution in the IV bag, or, most commonly, mixed in a minibag. The minibag is attached to what is an add-a-line or secondary medication administration set.

7. Transcribing IV orders follows the basic steps outlined in Chapter 16. The IV order must include the solution, the rate, and the start date. You would note any related nursing responsibilities or specific criteria, including site assessment and changing the IV and tubing. Orders for the same solution may sometimes be written in several ways. Be sure you understand the order that you are transcribing. Always check the rate carefully as well. Too much fluid, or the incorrect fluid, can be harmful, even fatal. Any medications given are recorded on a MAR. Medications given in minibags are usually recorded as scheduled medications. Those in solution in the main bag may be recorded on the scheduled MAR, or a medication infusion record.

8. Blood and blood products are ordered for anemia or excessive loss of blood and as a precaution for surgery. The most commonly ordered product is packed cells. A client's blood type and Rh factor must be checked carefully against donor blood to find a match and prevent potentially fatal reactions.

PROCEDURES		
MNEMONIC	NAME	ORDER CHECKED
NPO	NOTHING BY MOUTH	
FF	FULL FLUIDS	
CF	CLEAR FLUIDS	
PE	PUREE	
MN	MINCED	
REG	FULL DIET	
DD	DIABETIC DIET	
GF	GLUTEN FREE DIET	
LR	LOW RESIDUE	
SS	SURGICAL SOFT	
HP	HIGH PROTEIN	
HF	HIGH FIBRE	
EF	ENTERAL FEEDS	
PAR	PARENTERAL FEEDS	
BRAT	BANANA, RICE, APPLE, TOAST	
T&A	T&A (tonsillectomy and adenoidectomy) DIET- NO RED JELLO, HOT BEVERAGES	

Figure 18.2 Computerized diet look-up table.

Orders for Discharged Clients

You need to cancel meals for discharged clients. Find out when the client plans to leave. As discussed in Chapter 14, clients are encouraged to leave midmorning, so you need to notify Dietary to cancel lunch, using your facility's normal procedure. In some facilities, a formal discharge includes notifying Dietary. In computerized settings, the transcribed discharge order is automatically sent to Dietary, and lunch is usually cancelled automatically. However, if the discharge order comes through late, you need to call Dietary. Also, if a client has arranged to stay through lunch, you have to call Dietary and ask them to send the client's lunch up.

Diet Orders Related to Tests and Procedures

Diagnostic Tests

If the client is scheduled for a diagnostic test, you often need to ensure that diet has been appropriately altered. The diet preparation will not usually be spelled out in the order for the test; you will be expected to know what tests require diet restrictions and to make sure they are implemented. Before any test requiring an anesthetic, the client must remain NPO, usually for 8 to 10 hours. The same holds true for any test that involves visualizing parts of the gastrointestinal tract and for certain blood tests. Other dietary preparations may also apply. Consult the procedure or laboratory manual for clarification.

Barium Enema

Protocols vary for preparing clients for this test. Some doctors order a fibre-restricted noon meal the day before the test, followed by a clear fluid supper. Others require a full-fluid, low-fibre diet the whole day prior to the test. Still others have the client consume a special supplement up to two days prior to the test. Put the client's existing diet orders on hold, and initiate the preparatory diet orders. Make sure that the Dietary

Department is aware of the changes. In some computerized environments, the Dietary Department is notified that a client is having a barium enema and automatically adjusts the diet. In some facilities, you must post a sign at the client's bedside about diet changes; for example, it might read "clear fluids" or "NPO."

Cholecystography

This is a test to visualize the gallbladder. There is some controversy about meals the evening before. Some facilities restrict this meal; many, however, have dropped any restrictions on the basis of evidence that the evening meal does not affect test results. The client consumes a contrast medium 10 to 14 hours before the test and then fasts until the test is completed. Cancel or delay the client's breakfast, depending on the scheduled test time.

Glucose Tolerance Tests

The most common test in this category is the oral glucose tolerance test (OGTT). This test, used to diagnose diabetes, assesses the body's ability to use glucose by measuring blood glucose levels at specified intervals after the person has ingested a glucose solution. The client should be on a normal carbohydrate diet (at least 150 g per day) for at least three days before the test, and then remain NPO for 10 to 14 hours before the test. You or the nurse would post an NPO notice by the client's bedside. Delay or cancel breakfast on the morning of the test. The client must not eat, drink coffee or tea, or smoke after drinking the glucose solution until the test is finished.

Vanillylmandelic Acid Test (VMA)

This is a test involving a 24-hour urine collection (see Chapter 6), used to diagnose a disorder called pheochromocytoma. For 24 to 48 hours before the collection starts, the client must avoid coffee, tea, raisins, citrus fruits and juices, tomatoes, asparagus, alcohol, and vanilla. Make sure the appropriate diet is ordered.

Blood Tests

If a client is to have a fasting blood sugar or a blood test for cholesterol and triglycerides, he must remain NPO for 8 to 12 hours, except possibly for sips of water with certain medications. Post an NPO sign by the client's bed the night before. Usually, the blood will be drawn early in the morning just before breakfast arrives, and so you may have to hold breakfast briefly but will not usually need to cancel it. Clients who are aware that they are not to eat and are cognitively normal can be trusted to wait but should be reminded. If there is any doubt, the client should not be given the breakfast tray until after the blood is drawn.

Postoperative Diets

What and how soon the client is able to eat after surgery will depend on the type and extent of the surgery and the client's response to the anesthetic. General anesthetics cause the gastrointestinal tract to be sluggish and unable to digest food properly; some people recover intestinal motility faster than others. In addition, some people suffer nausea and vomiting. Physicians will consider the client's response in ordering postoperative diets. Clients who have had surgery on the gastrointestinal tract itself may be NPO for a period of time after the operation and often have nasogastric or **gastric suction**. Clients who have had minor surgery or local anesthetic are more likely to be able to eat later on the day of surgery but still may require a lighter than normal diet.

When a client comes back from the OR, the physician typically orders "CF to DAT" (meaning a progressive diet starting with clear fluids and progressing to a regular

GASTRIC SUCTION gentle suction applied to a tube placed in the stomach to remove excessive secretions, such as saliva and gastric juices, that tend to accumulate in the stomach after surgery or trauma because the intestine is sluggish. This can prevent or relieve nausea and vomiting.

diet as tolerated) or "Sips to DAT" (meaning starting with ice chips or sips only and progressing to a regular diet). Occasionally, a doctor will just write "as tolerated," leaving the progression of the diet up to the nurses. The nurses will let you know what type of diet to order for the client or will order it themselves.

Usually, a client who has just returned from the OR will be given only ice chips or sips of water. If the client has had major bowel surgery, even ice chips may not be allowed until **bowel sounds are present (BSP)**. The postoperative diet would advance then to clear fluids, full fluids, soft, and finally a regular diet. Table 18.2 shows the typical progression. However, the rate of return to a normal diet depends on the client and the surgery. Some clients may be able to omit certain steps. A client who has had a minor operation may have clear fluids for the first few hours and then move right on to a soft or regular diet. Some will take longer, especially if the surgery involves the gastrointestinal tract.

BOWEL SOUNDS PRESENT (BSP)   the audible return of gastrointestinal movement or function, also called peristalsis.

Postoperative Orders for Same-Day Admissions

You need to notify the Dietary Department about postoperative diets, but you cannot do so until the client comes to the client-care unit and the doctor writes the orders. Some hospitals have a standard protocol; if the client stays overnight but the surgery is minor, a soft diet might be ordered. For other surgeries, the diet could be clear fluids. If you get orders well ahead of time, you can simply send a manual or electronic requisition, but if you are processing orders close to a meal time and the client needs a tray, call Dietary. They may not get the requisition or check for new orders in time.

Postoperative Orders for Clients Already in Hospital

Sometimes, surgery is booked for a client already in hospital. Suppose Mr. Black had been admitted for investigation of abdominal pain. Three days later, his doctor discovered a tumour and decided to operate. As soon as you receive the operative orders and have a confirmed surgery date, cancel the client's diet, effective after dinner the day before surgery (or, otherwise, as ordered). Otherwise, breakfast will appear the next morning for Mr. Black, who is perhaps already in the OR, and the tray will be wasted. (Most facilities have strict rules that unused trays are to be returned untouched. They are not meant to provide snacks for hospital employees or visitors.) If the order comes in just before it needs to be implemented, call Dietary. In the two hours before a meal, they are too busy to check their computers or requisition forms.

Tube Feedings/Enteral Feeds

An **enteral feed** is one that is administered directly by a tube into the gastrointestinal system. Tube feedings bypass a person's swallowing mechanism and carry food directly into the stomach or bowel. They are used for individuals who cannot swallow, such as some stroke victims or people who have had part of their upper gastrointestinal tract removed because of cancer or trauma, and for people who cannot digest food (sometimes called malabsorption syndrome). Tubes may be inserted temporarily or permanently.

ENTERAL FEED   feeding by tube directly into the gastrointestinal system.

Table 18.2	Typical Progressive Diet after Major Surgery (not involving the GI tract)
Surgical day	NPO or ice chips or "sips" of water
Day one	Clear fluids.......maybe full fluids at suppertime
Day two	Full fluids.........maybe a soft diet at suppertime
Day three	Soft diet to a regular diet

Sites of Insertion

Tubes are usually referred to and ordered by site of insertion. Physicians often have preferences.

NASOGASTRIC TUBE (N-G TUBE or LEVINE TUBE) a feeding tube put through the nose into the stomach.

GASTROSTOMY TUBE (G-TUBE) a feeding tube inserted through an incision in the abdomen into the stomach.

JEJUNOSTOMY TUBE (J-TUBE) a feeding tube placed through the abdominal wall into the small bowel.

PERCUTANEOUS ENDOSCOPIC GASTROSTOMY TUBE (PEG TUBE, PEG CATHETER) a feeding tube inserted via endoscopy into the stomach or jejunum.

BARD BUTTON (MIC DEVICE) a feeding device placed permanently in the stomach to facilitate supplemental feedings.

◆ A **nasogastric tube** (**N-G tube**, or **Levine tube**) (see Figure 18.3) is put through the nose into the stomach. (*Gastric* means "relating to the stomach.") (A tube can also be inserted through the mouth into the stomach. Mouth tubes are rarely used in adults because they are uncomfortable and stimulate the gag reflex. They are more often used with young infants, who have weak gag reflexes and initially breathe only through the nose.) (Note: Levine tubes are also used to decompress the stomach, irrigate the stomach and treat as bleeding.)

◆ **Gastrostomy tubes** (**G-tubes**) are inserted through an incision in the abdomen into the stomach.

◆ **Jejunostomy tubes** (**J-tubes**) are placed through the abdominal wall into the jejunum, or small bowel. This site is chosen when the stomach cannot tolerate food because of such conditions as gastritis (inflammation of the stomach), pancreatitis (inflammation of the pancreas), or gastroesophageal reflux.

◆ Tubes can be inserted into the duodenum, but this is not common.

◆ A **percutaneous endoscopic gastrostomy tube** (**PEG tube** or **catheter**) (see Figure 18.4) is inserted through a puncture through the skin and subcutaneous tissues of the abdomen and stomach using an endoscope (a flexible instrument used to visualize organs). This catheter or tube has a bulb that is inflated once inside the stomach or jejunum and keeps the tube from falling out.

◆ A **Bard button** or **MIC device** is surgically implanted in the stomach to facilitate supplemental feedings. The Bard button is made of pliable silicone, with a mushroom-shaped dome at one end and a flat rectangular flap with a safety plug on the abdominal side. Only the flap with the safety plug attached is visible on the skin surface of the abdomen. An anti-reflux valve helps prevent gastric leakage through the tube. Special feeding tubes are necessary to connect the button to a feeding bag or syringe. The MIC key is also made of pliable silicone, with a contoured disc on the abdominal surface and an anti-reflux valve, and requires a special feeding set to connect to a feeding bag or syringe.

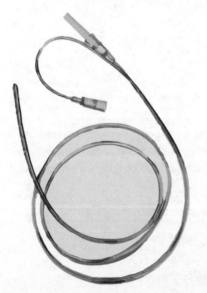

Figure 18.3   Levine tube.

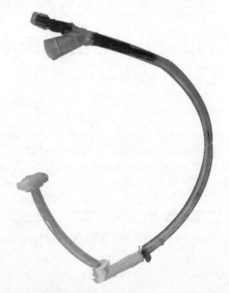

Figure 18.4   PEG tube.

Orders Relating to GI Surgery and Procedures

If a client has gastrointestinal surgery, the nurses monitor the status and progress of gastrointestinal function closely, including the return of normal motility and normal elimination patterns. Interventions are usually needed until function is re-established and doctors issue orders related to nursing care and assessments. The following are some of the more common gastrointestinal surgeries.

Bowel Resection, Colostomy, and Ileostomy

A **bowel resection** and **anastomosis** (may also be called **end-to-end anastomosis**) involves removing a section of the bowel and connecting the healthy ends together again. This can occur anywhere along the large or small bowel. If the bowel cannot be reconnected to the rectal portion because it is diseased, a **colostomy** or an **ileostomy** will be created. This is a procedure wherein the end of the bowel is brought out to the abdomen and a **stoma**, or artificial opening, is created, through which feces are excreted (Figure 19.7). A colostomy involves the colon or large bowel; an ileostomy involves the ileum or distal small bowel. Conditions that necessitate a colostomy or ileostomy include cancer, ulcerative colitis, and Crohn's disease. In the case of a colostomy, the fecal matter has been largely processed, and a formed stool is produced; in the case of an ileostomy, fluid has not been absorbed, and the result is an almost continuous drainage of loose fecal matter.

Colostomy and Ileostomy Supplies

A wide range of equipment is used for clients who have colostomies or ileostomies. Disposable or reusable bags, shown in Figure 19.8, collect the waste. They are attached with "wafers," devices that fit around the stoma, or opening. The wafers have an adhesive back and stick to the abdomen, forming a seal around the stoma. The ostomy bag attaches to the wafer, also forming a seal. Doctor's orders do not usually refer to ostomy supplies, but a nurse may ask you to order them.

BOWEL RESECTION (ANASTOMOSIS or END-TO-END ANASTOMOSIS)   surgery wherein a section of bowel is removed, and the remaining bowel is reconnected.

COLOSTOMY   a surgical procedure that creates an artificial opening from the colon to the surface of the abdomen, through which feces are excreted.

ILEOSTOMY   a surgical procedure that creates an artificial opening from the ileum to the surface of abdomen, through which feces are excreted.

STOMA   an artificial opening, in this case, one from the bowel through the abdominal wall.

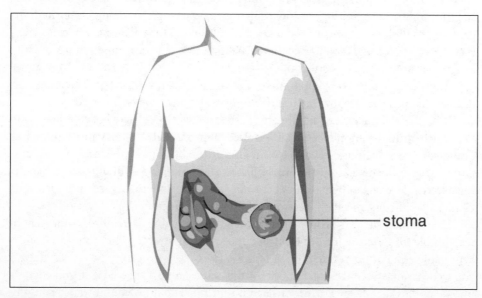

Figure 19.7   A stoma.

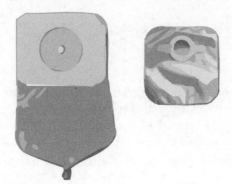

Figure 19.8   Ostomy bag and wafer.

Bowel Irrigations

Bowel irrigation may be ordered if a client with a colostomy is having difficulty pass-ing stool. It is based on the same principle as an enema or an evacuation suppository. Fluid is introduced into the bowel through an irrigation tube placed into the stoma. Bowel irrigation trays or kits are available from Central Supply.

Nasogastric Suction

Nasogastric suction involves inserting a tube through the nose into the stomach and using an electric suction device to gently remove solids, liquids, or gases from the stomach or small intestine. It may be short term or long term.

Following surgery on the GI tract or related organs (e.g., removal of the gallblad-der through a large incision), nasogastric suction is frequently necessary to rest the bowel and/or allow it to heal. It may also be ordered to relieve excessive nausea and vomiting, as occurs in some pregnant women, to obtain a sample of gastric contents for testing, or to empty the stomach prior to gastric surgery. Suction may also be ordered as conservative treatment to decompress the stomach or small intestine when a bowel obstruction is suspected.

Various suction machines are available, most of them portable ones brought to the client's room. A popular device is the Gomco machine (illustrated in Figure 19.9), an electric pump that gives intermittent suction by varying the air pressure. Red and green lights flash as the pressure changes, indicating that the suction is working. There is also a switch for high and low suction. The high setting is rarely used. If the doctor's order does not specify, low suction is assumed.

Another type of suction apparatus is a portable electric motor. Some facilities have devices that provide negative suction from the wall beside the client's bed.

Regardless of the type of suction, the gastric material is collected in a drainage bot-tle, which must be monitored and emptied appropriately. Nurses must record all drainages. Some facilities leave space for this at the bottom of the vital signs graph. Others record the data as output under Tubes and Drains on a fluid balance sheet. In the electronic environment, nurses usually enter it under Nursing Interventions, Clinical Paremeters, or on an electronic fluid balance document.

If a Gomco suction or any other type of suction unit is required, you may be responsible for ordering it from Central Supply. Nasogastric (Levine) tubes are usually kept in the clean utility room. If none of the correct size is available, the nurses may ask you to order one from Central Supply (or the equivalent). If they need it immediately, phone and arrange to pick it up or have it sent up. The lift or dumbwaiter could be

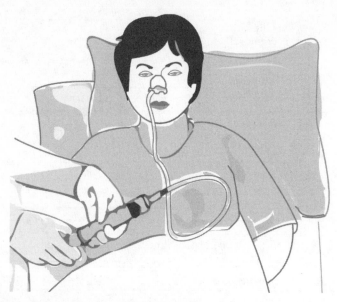

Figure 19.9   Nasogastric tube with Gomco suction.

used for this purpose. As discussed in Chapter 18, nasogastric (Levine) tubes comes in a variety of sizes. The most common sizes used for nasogastric suction in adults are 16 or 19 Fr. The physician may not order a specific size, leaving it up to the nurses' judgment. When you phone Central Supply, specify the type and size of tube you need.

Another type of tube, a sump tube, may be used for gastric lavage.

Suction Orders

Doctors ordering suction may be specific about type or may leave details to be assumed. A doctor may order "Insert nasogastric tube to Gomco suction drainage." When suction is not specifically ordered as continuous, it is assumed to be intermittent, so the doctor may simply order "Gomco suction." Or, he may not even specify the type, but just order "NG suction."

In this case, you would assume that he wants whatever type of suction is most commonly used in your facility. If the nurses are unclear about the type of suction or pattern of suction wanted, they can ask the doctor for clarification.

Suction orders are usually transcribed to the kardex or PI screen. Figure 19.10 shows a kardex with an order transcribed for a nasogastric tube with Gomco suction to gastric drainage. In this format, the order is transcribed under a heading for Tubes and Drains. Note that an order for a rectal tube PRN is also transcribed under this section. An order to keep the client NPO is transcribed under Diet.

Sometimes, the NG tube is inserted in the OR, in which case there may be no related insertion orders. The order may say "NG suction to straight drainage," indicating that it is already in place. This would be transcribed in the same manner onto the electronic or traditional kardex along with any assessments.

Trays for NG Tube Irrigation

If an NG tube becomes plugged, it must be rinsed or irrigated with normal saline to clear the obstruction. The nurse detaches the NG tube from the tube leading to the suction machine and, with a large syringe, instills a measured amount of saline or water into the tube leading into the client's stomach. The nurse either withdraws the fluid with the syringe or simply reconnects the NG tube to the suction machine; the

Diet: Type/Texture:	Clip/suture Removal:					
NPO						
Self:	Intake/output Record					
With assist:						
	Tubes/drains					
	N/G tube to Gomco					
	Rectal tube					
	PRN					

Figure 19.10   Kardex showing suction order.

fluid then drains into the large bottle at the other end of the suction tubing. The nurses may keep a tray at the client's bedside containing the apparatus needed to irrigate or flush the tubing. They may ask you to order an irrigation tray. It is important to specify the type of irrigation tray needed; a bladder irrigation tray, for example, is quite different from an NG irrigation tray.

The Urinary System

The urinary tract, shown in Figure 19.11, consists of two kidneys, two ureters, the urinary bladder, and the urethra. (This system is often referred to as the genitourinary [GU] tract because it shares structures with the genital organs.) The urinary system removes waste from the body in the form of urine; it works with other body systems, such as the lungs, the intestines, and the integumentary system. Urine is produced in

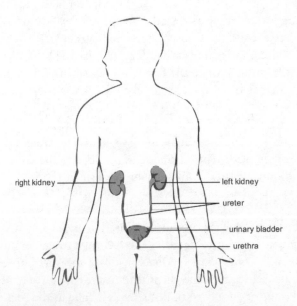

Figure 19.11   The urinary tract.

problems. Anything that interferes with the exchange of oxygen and carbon dioxide will cause trouble breathing.

For the lungs to function optimally, the following factors must be present:

- Adequate levels of oxygen in the air
- Clear airways so that air movement is not obstructed or diminished
- Strong respiratory muscles to facilitate inhalation and expiration
- Lungs able to expand and contract adequately to draw in sufficient air
- Adequate blood supply to the lungs
- Adequate circulation and hemoglobin levels to transport oxygen to all parts of the body

Problems in any of these areas will lead to decreased oxygenation. If oxygenation is decreased sharply enough, clinical signs will become evident on assessment, and laboratory and diagnostic tests will show abnormal results.

Conditions That Affect Oxygenation

Many conditions affect oxygenation, some of them not directly related to the respiratory system. The most common direct causes of breathing problems are viral or bacterial **pneumonia** (an acute infection of the lungs), **asthma**, and chronic lung conditions, such as **emphysema**, a degeneration of the alveolar sacs, and **chronic obstructive lung disease (COLD)**, also known as **chronic obstructive pulmonary disease (COPD)**. Because the cardiovascular system and the respiratory system are interdependent, heart problems also generally affect oxygenation. **Hemorrhage** and surgery can also cause **hypoxia**.

Health Professionals Involved with Respiratory Problems

Respiratory problems are treated and assessed by a team that includes the physician, the respiratory technologist, the nurse, and the physiotherapist. While their work may overlap, most facilities use a coordinated team approach to carry out physicians' orders and provide feedback on the clients' progress.

Registered Respiratory Technologist

Registered respiratory technologists (RTs) are trained to recognize and treat clients with respiratory difficulties. They may initiate, administer, and supervise treatments ordered by the doctor, respond to cardiac arrests, and supervise oxygen therapy devices, such as inhalation devices and respirators. They work closely with the client, the nurses, the family doctors, and the specialists on both client care and specialty units. They also administer and evaluate the results of related tests, for example, the pulmonary function test (PFT) and blood gases.

Physiotherapist

Physiotherapists (sometimes referred to simply as "physio," a short form that also describes physiotherapy) provide respiratory assessments and related physiotherapy. When a doctor orders "chest physio," the physiotherapists assess clients, devise and help with deep breathing exercises, and teach them how to cough effectively to keep the lungs clear.

PNEUMONIA an acute infection of the tissues of the lung.

ASTHMA a disease that affects the air passages in the lung, causing wheezing and shortness of breath.

HEMORRHAGE loss of a large amount of blood (greater than 500 cc for an average adult).

EMPHYSEMA a disease characterized by gradual destruction of the alveoli, which fuse to form larger air spaces. Exchange of oxygen and carbon dioxide through these larger air sacs is inadequate.

CHRONIC OBSTRUCTIVE LUNG DISEASE (COLD) or CHRONIC OBSTRUCTIVE PULMONARY DISEASE (COPD) any chronic lung condition in which the flow of expired air is slowed down.

HYPOXIA insufficient oxygen in blood or tissue.

Nurse

Nursing staff provide ongoing assessment and feedback about a client's oxygenation status. If an RT or physiotherapist is not available, a nurse can initiate and supervise chest physio or administer oxygen and inhalation treatments.

Orders Related to Oxygenation
Chest Physiotherapy

Chest physio is often ordered for clients with a build-up of secretions in the lungs. Techniques vary from routines clients can do on their own to interventions provided by physiotherapists or the nurses.

Deep Breathing and Coughing Exercises

Secretions in the lungs can become thick and difficult for the client to cough up. If the secretions are left sitting in the lungs, they can become infected or exacerbate an already present infection, further compromising the client's breathing. Many clients can cough these secretions up by themselves if they are shown the proper technique. Either a physiotherapist or a nurse can teach the client deep breathing and coughing exercises (DB&C), which should usually be done every two to three hours while awake. Often, a physiotherapist and a nurse work together to ensure that the client understands the exercises and performs them properly and regularly. A device called a spirometer (discussed later) may help the client assess how effectively she is breathing and performing the exercises. Doctors often order DB&C for clients with respiratory difficulties.

Chest Physio with Postural Drainage

People with large amounts of mucus or thick secretions or who have weak breathing muscles or ineffective coughs may need more than DB&C to loosen and move the secretions out of the lungs. They may be helped by chest physio accompanied by **postural drainage**, that is, positioning the client with her head lower than her body so that gravity can help move the secretions. The physiotherapist may also manually loosen stubborn chest secretions by **clapping** (also called **percussion**): using cupped hands to gently but firmly strike affected regions of the chest to move secretions to the bronchi, from where they can be coughed up more easily. She may also stimulate movement of secretions by placing flattened hands over the congested area and using rapid **vibrations**.

Orders for Chest Physiotherapy

When doctors order chest physio, orders may be more or less specific, as in the following examples:

> Chest physio bid
>
> Encourage DB&C exercises q2h while awake
>
> Postural drainage by physio tid
>
> Routine post-op physio by physiotherapist

If the doctor orders simply "chest physio bid," the order implies a request for an assessment and development of an appropriate routine. Send a requisition (paper or electronic) to the Physiotherapy Department. Transcribe these orders to the kardex or PI screen, either under Respiratory or under Treatments or Interventions.

A doctor might specifically order, for example, "Encourage DB&C exercises q2h while awake." This order can be initiated and supervised by the physiotherapist or the

POSTURAL DRAINAGE
positioning the client with the head lower than the body so that gravity can help drain the mucus and secretions.

CLAPPING or PERCUSSION
using cupped hands to gently but firmly strike affected regions of the chest to move secretions.

VIBRATIONS rapid movements of flattened hands over the client's chest to move secretions.

nurse and does not require a requisition. On many surgical units, a physiotherapist or nurse routinely visits all postoperative clients, with or without an order, to implement these exercises, either routinely or if they are having trouble breathing. The physiotherapist may complete an initial assessment and run through the exercises with the client once or twice. The nurses encourage the client to continue with the exercises and complete chess assessments as per protocol. If sustained contact with the physiotherapist is required, usually an order and a requisition are necessary.

If a doctor orders "postural drainage by physio tid," this would require a requisition because it is more than the routine treatment. TID would probably involve a morning–afternoon–evening routine or a morning–early afternoon–late afternoon routine. Add the times to the kardex or PI screen; typical times for this order would be 1000, 1400, and 1700; or 1000, 1600, and 2000. If there is no physiotherapist on duty in the evening, the nurses would complete the postural drainage routine.

If the facility does not have physiotherapists to routinely see post-op clients, the nurses would recommend a physio consult if they deemed it necessary. A doctor may also order a consult, perhaps as "Routine post-op physio by physiotherapist." The therapist will visit the client, assess his needs, and implement a specific routine. If a formal request is made, send a requisition to the Physiotherapy Department. Physiotherapy is often part of a client's discharge planning.

Nursing Assessment

Vital Signs/Respiratory Assessments

Respiratory rate is part of routine vital signs assessment (along with temperature and pulse), normally done at least once or twice a day (see Chapter 16). Nurses will also assess other characteristics of the client's breathing, such as depth and regularity. Vital signs also provide an indication of the cardiac condition. Blood pressure is not a routine part of vital signs but may be added on request. Vital signs are usually taken more frequently for postoperative clients until they are stable and for clients with abnormal vital signs, such as an elevated temperature, pulse, or respiratory rate, perhaps accompanied by dyspnea. Nurses may increase the frequency of vital signs within policy guidelines if their assessments indicate a problem, or the doctor may order a certain frequency. For example, a doctor may order one of the following:

V/S QID

V/S and BP QID

V/S q15 min × 4, q1/2h × 6, q1h × 8 and then QID if stable

In the last example, the doctor wants signs checked every 15 minutes for an hour, then every half-hour for three hours, followed by every hour for eight hours. After that, if the vital signs are stable, the nurses can reduce assessment to four times a day.

If the doctor is concerned about a client's blood pressure or circulation, she may issue more specific orders for blood pressure assessments. For example, "Monitor BP in lying and sitting position, in both arms bid."

The doctor orders blood pressure to be read with the patient in two different positions to see if it changes with position. If so, the client may be suffering postural hypotension, that is, an abnormally low blood pressure in certain positions. Taking blood pressure in both arms will pick up compromised circulation on one side, for example, because of a narrowed artery.

Chest Assessments

In a chest assessment, a doctor, respiratory technician, or more usually a nurse, assesses the client's colour and ease of breathing and auscultates or listens to the client's lungs through a stethoscope. If breath sounds are diminished or absent, that indicates impeded or diminished air exchange caused by such conditions as pneumonia. Adventitious or extra sounds include **crackles**, or **crepitation**, and **rhonchi** (singular, rhonchus), or **wheezes**. Crepitation sounds something like air blown through a straw immersed in fluid and usually indicates the presence of fluid in the small airways. Rhonchi can be high pitched or low pitched and are caused by air moving through airways narrowed by swelling or partial obstruction.

Chest assessments (CA) are routine for postoperative clients and for those with cardiorespiratory problems. The physician may order a chest assessment at specific intervals or may rely on hospital routines. A respiratory unit might have qid as routine, whereas an orthopedic unit might have bid or od as routine. Postoperative chest assessments range from bid to qid and decrease as the client recovers. Transcribe the order to the kardex or PI screen under Oxygenation or Nursing Assessments/Interventions and add the times; for assessments od, you would probably record the time as 1000. No requisition is required.

Diagnostic Tests for Oxygenation

Pulse Oximetry

Pulse oximetry is a method used by nurses and respiratory therapists to determine oxygen levels in red blood cells in the arterial blood. A pulse oximeter, shown in Figure 20.3, is a sensor that can be attached to the client's finger, toe, or sometimes the earlobe. One part of the sensor emits two lights, one of which is a specific frequency of red. The red light is absorbed by oxygenated hemoglobin, and the other is absorbed by deoxygenated hemoglobin. On the other side of the oximeter, a photodetector reads the amount of light absorbed by oxygenated and deoxygenated hemoglobin. The proportion of hemoglobin that is carrying oxygen is an indicator of respiratory status. The measurement is reported as arterial blood oxygen saturation (SaO_2 or O_2 Sat). Normal adult SaO_2 values should be at least 95 percent.

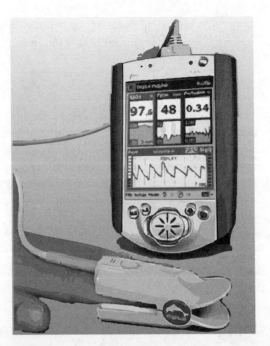

Figure 20.3   Pulse oximeter.

cancelling or delaying meals and ensuring that the nurses know that the client will be NPO the night before the procedure. A consent is required for this procedure.

Cardiac Catheterization

Also called a "heart cath" or an angiogram (see Figure 20.11), this procedure is performed in a special lab. A thin wire called a cardiac catheter is inserted through an artery, usually in the thigh, and threaded into the heart. A dye is injected, and X-rays are taken of the arteries. The client usually requires some sedation. Smaller hospitals may not offer this test, and so the client may have to be transported to a larger hospital. Book the appointment at the appropriate facility, and then implement the preparation for the client. Send the client's chart and MAR along with him. Most facilities require the client be NPO the night before the procedure. A consent is necessary.

				McCarthy, Carolyn 588 Church St. Halifax N.S, B3M 9G9 F 12 10 41 082399 454923766 Sokolov, Dr. I.
	ECG stat			
	Portable Chest X-ray PA and lateral			
	Transfer to Telemetry for 48 hrs.			
	Book for angiogram this week			
	Arrange for pacemaker insertion in OR Friday			
Date Sept 1 /04	Time	Physician's Name Printed Dr. Sokolov	Physician's signature Dr. I. Sokolov	

Figure 20.11   Order for cardiac assessments and interventions.

Cardiopulmonary Emergencies

You need to be alert to the possibility of cardiac or respiratory arrests and know what you have to do if one occurs.

Respiratory Arrest

A respiratory arrest occurs as a result of a decreased ability to breathe adequately or a partial or complete airway obstruction. When a person loses consciousness, his tongue may obstruct the airway. Another common cause of obstruction is choking on food or vomitus. This risk is the reason individuals who are going for surgery are kept NPO for eight to 12 hours before the operation. If there is food in the client's upper GI tract and the client vomits, the vomitus could be aspirated into the lung and cause a respiratory arrest. Spasm or edema of the vocal cords, inflammation, and trauma can also precipitate a respiratory arrest. A respiratory arrest is often anticipated with a high-risk delivery, and a respiratory therapist as well as additional medical staff may be in attendance. As part of transcribing these orders, Mary would call the technician to do the ECG STAT, print the requisitions on the floor, call Radiology to do the x-ray, print the requisition on the floor, and arrange for the required tests. Consent would be needed for the angiogram and the pacemaker insertion.

Cardiac Arrest

A cardiac arrest is one of the most urgent medical emergencies and frequently results in death. A cardiac arrest may result from a mechanical failure of the heart or a failure of the heart's electrical conduction system. Because the circulatory system interacts so closely with the respiratory system, these failures may result in either cardiac or respiratory arrest. If not immediately treated, both cardiac and respiratory systems will stop working. Consent would be needed for the angiogram and the pacemaker insertion.

Calling an Arrest

If a cardiac or respiratory arrest occurs, you must "call the arrest," that is, notify the appropriate people. Know the procedures and codes for cardiac and respiratory arrests; in some facilities, the same code is used for both; other facilities use two different codes. Act quickly, but remain calm. Collect the required information, usually the client's room and bed numbers—make sure you have the correct numbers. Most facilities have a special emergency number. Go to the nearest telephone and dial the number. Give the information clearly and concisely to the operator. Response will be swift.

Summary

1. The cardiovascular and respiratory systems work independently and interdependently to maintain adequate amounts of oxygen in the blood. Any condition that affects one system will affect the client's oxygenation and may also affect other systems. Clients who are admitted with respiratory or cardiovascular conditions and postoperative clients will likely be monitored for oxygenation status.

2. Respiratory therapists, physiotherapists, and nurses provide ongoing assessment and care related to respiratory problems.

3. The purpose of chest physio is to assist with the removal of secretions from the lungs. Clients are taught deep breathing and coughing exercises (DB&C). Physiotherapists may manually loosen secretions by clapping or vibrating. Postural drainage uses gravity by positioning the head lower than the body.

4. Respiratory assessment (rate, rhythm, volume, etc.) (see Appendix) is done as part of routine vital signs assessment. Chest assessments, completed by nurses, respiratory therapists, and physiotherapists, involve auscultating for abnormal sounds, such as crackles (crepitation) and wheezes (rhonchi). Chest assessment (CA) is routine for postoperative clients and may be ordered with specific frequency.

5. Pulse oximetry uses a small light-sensing device to determine oxygen saturation; it may be ordered as continuous or intermittent. A peak flowmeter measures the flow of air out of the lungs. Arterial blood gases (ABG) measure the levels of oxygen and carbon dioxide in blood and the pH level. They are often ordered stat. For a stat order, keep the requisition on the floor until the sample is taken. Report ABG results promptly. Sputum samples may be taken for culture and sensitivity or cytology. Pulmonary function tests are usually done in the Respiratory Department and require a requisition.

6. Incentive spirometers encourage clients' deep breathing exercises. Inhalation therapy is often used to treat asthma. Oxygen therapy is commonly ordered postoperatively and for clients who do not have enough blood oxygen. Oxygen may be given through nasal prongs (NP) or by face mask. Oxygen orders may be continuous or prn; they specify concentration, method of delivery, and volume per minute. Observe safety measures around oxygen. Ventilators help clients who cannot adequately breathe independently. They are most frequently seen in intensive care units. A tracheostomy is an artificial opening in the throat through which a tube is inserted to help with breathing.

7. Clients who are unable to cough up secretions by themselves may be suctioned. Suctioning through the nose and mouth reaches the back of the mouth and throat. Deep suctioning involves the bronchi. Endotracheal suctioning goes through an endotracheal or tracheostomy tube and is a strictly sterile procedure.

8. Orders relating to the cardiovascular system often overlap with those relating to respiratory assessments. Vital signs, chest assessments, and chest X-rays relate to both systems. In doing a peripheral vascular assessment (PVA), a nurse checks skin colour and temperature, pulse, and sensation. A chest X-ray is usually ordered as AP and Lateral,

specifying front, back, and side views. It may be ordered as a portable if the client cannot move to Radiology. An ECG (or EKG) measures the heart's electrical activity and is one of the most commonly ordered cardiovascular tests. Variations include a stress test and a Holter monitor, which provides continuous monitoring. In cardiac catheterization (angiogram), a dye is injected and X-rays of arteries are taken.

9. Pacemakers are inserted to regulate the heartbeat through electrical signals; insertion is an operative procedure.

10. A respiratory arrest or a cardiac arrest is an emergency. You must know your responsibility and how to call the arrest. Act swiftly, make sure you have the correct information, and remain calm.

Key Terms

ARRHYTHMIA 532	CONGESTIVE HEART FAILURE	HYPOXIA 533
ARTERIES 529	(CHF) 531	ISCHEMIA 545
ARTERIOLES 529	CRASH CART 531	MYOCARDIAL INFARCT 531
ARTERIOSCLEROSIS 531	CRACKLES (CREPITATION) 536	NASOPHARYNGEAL SUCTIONING
ASTHMA 533	CYANOSIS 545	544
ATHEROSCLEROSIS 531	DEEP SUCTIONING 544	OROPHARYNGEAL SUCTIONING
ATRIAL FIBRILLATION 532	DIASTOLIC PRESSURE 531	544
BRADYCARDIA 546	DYSPNEA 532	PNEUMONIA 533
BRUIT 546	EMPHYSEMA 533	POSTURAL DRAINAGE 534
CANNULA 543	ENDOTRACHEAL SUCTIONING 544	RALES 536
CAPILLARIES 529	HEMATOCRIT 530	RHONCHI (WHEEZES) 536
CEREBRAL VASCULAR	HEMATOPOIESIS 529	SYSTOLIC PRESSURE 531
ACCIDENT 531	HEMOGLOBIN 530	TRACHEOSTOMY 543
CHRONIC OBSTRUCTIVE LUNG	HEMORRHAGE 533	VEINS 529
DISEASE 533	HYPERTENSION	VENULES 529
CIRCUMORAL PALLOR 545	(HIGH BLOOD PRESSURE) 531	VIBRATIONS 534
CLAPPING (PERCUSSION) 534		

Review Questions

1. What is the relationship between the cardiovascular and respiratory systems with respect to oxygenation?

2. List the main organs in the cardiovascular and respiratory systems.

3. State the role of hemoglobin in the oxygenation process.

4. What roles do respiratory therapists and physiotherapists play in respiratory assessment and care?

5. What is included in a chest assessment, and what is the purpose of this assessment?

6. What is the principle by which pulse oximetry works?

7. Why are blood gases sometimes ordered along with or instead of oximetry?

8. What is unique about an order for sputum for cytology or AFB?

9. Describe the purpose and use of the spirometer on the client-care unit.

10. What would you do if a client had a respiratory or cardiac arrest?

Application Exercises

1. Summarize the physiology and function of the respiratory and cardiovascular systems. Use a detailed diagram to illustrate the structure of each.

2. Research three common respiratory conditions and three common cardiovascular conditions. For each, describe the following:

   a. Common assessments used to diagnose and monitor the condition
   b. The etiology of the condition
   c. How it interferes with oxygenation

3. Mr. Loton is in hospital with CHF and SOB. He is weak and semiconscious.

   a. What is meant by the acronym SOB?
   b. What is meant by the acronym CHF?

   c. Why might Dr. Bobb have ordered suction after the client had chest physio?
   d. Briefly describe the function and purpose of the Venturi mask.
   e. Why were ABGs ordered based on O_2 sats from oximetry?
   f. What is meant by PA and lateral in the order for the chest X-ray?
   g. Why is a portable X-ray ordered in this case?
   h. Transcribe the orders in Figure 20.12 according to the protocol outlined by your professor.

	V/S quid x 48 then bid		**Loton, Walter**
	Chest physio quid suction after physio PRN		**477 Grange St.**
	Sputum for cytology x 3		**Acton, ON L7R 2R4**
	O_2 by Venturi mask @ 34%		**M 17 04 38 034902**
	Pulse ox quid. ABGs if sats drop below 92%		**2779453775**
	EKG in 2 days & chest X-ray PA and lateral stat portable		**Bobb, Dr. R.**
Date Sept 1 /04	Time	Physician's Name Printed Dr. Bobb	Physician's signature Dr. R. Bobb

Figure 20.12   Doctor's orders for Walter Loton.

Web Sites of Interest

The Respiratory System
http://www.stemnet.nf.ca/CITE/respiratory.htm

The Cardiovascular System, animated
http://www.innerbody.com/text/card03.html
http://www.innerbody.com/image/cardov.html
http://www.biologyinmotion.com/cardio/

Abnormal Breath Sounds
http://www.rnceus.com/resp/respabn.html

How to Use a Peak Flowmeter
http://www.caritas.ab.ca/ther_new/respcare/asthm
   a/peakflow.html

Spirometry Video
http://oac.med.jhmi.edu/res_phys/Encyclopedia/S
   pirometry/Spirometry.HTML

Web Sites of Interest

Explanation of Decubitus Ulcers or Pressure Sores
http://www.ldhpmed.com/DU_explanation.htm

Down-Under Wool
http://www.medicalsheepskins.com/bedsores2.
  htm

This site about sheepskins shows the stages of
development of a bedsore.

Understanding Patient Restraints—A Hospital's
Decision to Use Restraints
http://library.lp.findlaw.com/articles/file/00340/
  001457/title/subject/topic/health%20law_
  government%20regulation/filename/
  healthlaw_1_336

Regulations and Recommendations for the Use of
Chemical, Verbal, and Physical Restraints
http://intotem.buffnet.net/mhw/37APRestraints1.
  html

Activities of Daily Living: Tips for the Caregiver
http://www.seniornavigator.com/content/
  community/adls.asp

Mobility Devices
http://www.bragmanhealth.com/books/aging/
  ch08.html

Using Crutches and Canes
http://physicaltherapy.about.com/library/weekly/
  aa122699.htm

Safe Use of Wheelchairs
http://www.safety.uwa.edu.au/policies/
  use_of_wheelchairs

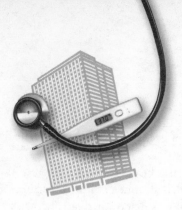

Vital Signs

Vital signs are measurements that serve as indicators of an individual's overall health. Signs routinely monitored include temperature, pulse, respiratory rate, and blood pressure.

Although they are not a vital sign, height and weight measurements (or **mensuration**) are also important. Weight gain or loss may indicate a pathological condition. Weight is also needed to determine dosage of medication or anesthesia. Mensuration is particularly important in assessing the growth and development of infants and children. Infant measurement includes not only weight and length but also head and sometimes chest circumferences. For children, these measurements are plotted on a growth chart. The child's growth can then be compared with "normal" parameters. This information is also used in conjunction with assessing the child's developmental milestones.

MENSURATION
measurement of height, weight, and infant head and sometimes chest circumferences.

Reasons for Taking Vital Signs

◆ *To screen for medical problems.* Taking signs routinely gives the provider a baseline so that significant changes can be noted and disease recognized early. For example, high blood pressure is often picked up at a routine screening.

◆ *To help the provider make a diagnosis.* Vital signs alone will rarely diagnose a condition but, in conjunction with other assessment information, can confirm or rule out a diagnosis.

◆ *To monitor a client's condition* and provide information the provider needs to modify treatment.

Vital signs are taken routinely for almost all hospitalized clients. Physicians will order which signs to take (e.g., some patients may not require blood pressure taken) and how often. In the physician's office, sign taking depends on the situation. Visits for minor complaints may not require vital signs. When infection is suspected, only temperature, pulse, and respirations may be taken. Complete vital signs are taken at a complete or annual physical examination and for clients being monitored for chronic problems such as heart disease, kidney disease, and hypertension.

Vital signs are sometimes monitored at home—by the client or a community nurse—particularly for clients with hypertensive disorders. In the health office, the nurse, physician, or HOP may measure vital signs.

Taking vital signs is not a regulated activity (as discussed in Chapter 1 and Chapter 15). In hospitals, nurses usually take vital signs, but a clinical secretary may sometimes do so. In doctors' offices, vital signs are commonly taken by doctors or nurses but may also be taken by a trained HOP. Remember that you are performing a technical act, recording, and reporting results. You should be aware of abnormal results that the doctor needs to know about immediately, but you are not qualified to interpret or diagnose.

Body Temperature

FEBRILE   involving fever.

Taking a client's temperature can indicate state of health, help diagnose **febrile** disease, and track response to treatment.

Body temperature is the balance between the heat body cells produce through metabolism and the heat the body loses to the environment through various mechanisms, such as the skin and through breathing. It is determined largely by a person's *basal metabolic rate* (BMR) (see Chapter 18). The hypothalamus, located at the base of the brain, acts as the body's "thermostat."

SURFACE TEMPERATURE   the temperature of the skin and fat.

CORE (INTERNAL) TEMPERATURE   the temperature of vital organs, such as the brain, heart, and liver.

The **surface temperature**—the temperature of the skin and fat—rises and falls in response to the environment. A more accurate indicator of actual body temperature is the **core (or internal) temperature**—the temperature of vital organs, such as the brain, heart and liver. This temperature is approximated by measurements in the ear, mouth, underarm, or rectum.

Reasons for Variation in Normal Temperature

- *Time of day (**diurnal variation or circadian cycle**):* A person's temperature may vary by up to 1 degree C over the day, with the lowest point typically between 0200 and 0600 and the highest point between 1700 and 2000.
- *Individual metabolic rate*
- *Age:* Children tend to have higher temperatures than do adults; elderly people tend to have lower temperatures than do younger adults. Temperatures are more labile (variable) in children and old people than in younger adults.
- *Environment:* Body temperature may vary somewhat with prolonged exposure to extreme temperatures or with over- or underdressing.

Table A.1 | Normal and Febrile Temperatures

Site	Average temperature Degrees C	Degrees F	Normal temperature range Degrees C	Degrees F	Fever: above Degrees C	Degrees F
oral	37	98.6	36.3 or 36.5–37.5 or 37.8	97.3 or 97.7–99.5 or 100	37.8 or 38	100 or 100.4
rectal	37.5	99.5	37–38	98.6–100.4	38	100.4
axillary	36.5	97.7	36–37	96.8–98.6	37.2	99
tympanic	37.5	99.5	36.3 or 36.5–37.5 or 37.8	97.3 or 97.7–99.5 or 100	37.8 or 38	100 or 100.4

1. Sources vary slightly in giving reference values.
2. Temperatures are normally taken in degrees Celsius. However, clients may think in Fahrenheit and may report temperatures taken at home in degrees Fahrenheit. (See Figure A.1.)

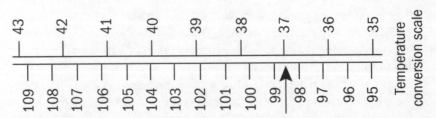

Figure A.1   Celsius–Fahrenheit conversion scale.

Precautions

◆ Try to ensure a quiet environment. (Noise may mask the reading and may disturb the client, altering the measurement.)

◆ If the client has just come in, ask about exercise. If the client has just exercised, wait 15 minutes.

◆ Never take blood pressure in an injured arm or in one where there is the known presence of a blocked blood vessel or any type of implanted device.

◆ If a reading shows an unexpected elevation, wait 10 to 15 minutes. Talk to the client and allow the client to rest, then retake the reading. Sometimes, the stress of a doctor visit can lead to elevated BP.

◆ Try not to show any facial or vocal reaction; if you look puzzled, surprised, or anxious, this will stress the client and could interfere with an accurate measurement.

◆ Keep the equipment in good repair. The unit should be calibrated routinely.

Key Terms

APICAL PULSE 570	FEBRILE 566	PYREXIA 567
CORE (INTERNAL) TEMPERATURE 566	HYPERTENSION 574	SURFACE TEMPERATURE 566
COUPLING 571	MENSURATION 565	
	PERIPHERAL PULSE 570	

GLOSSARY

ABSORPTION the process by which a medication is taken into the body, broken down, and transformed into a form that the body can use.

ACTIVE IMMUNITY immunity produced when the body makes its own antibodies in response to either natural exposure to a pathogen or artificial exposure through vaccination.

ACTIVE INFECTION an infection in which signs and symptoms are present.

ACUTE CARE care for a client who is acutely ill, that is, very ill, but with an illness expected to run a short course, (as opposed to a chronic illness). Acute care is provided for clients with a variety of health problems.

ACUTE INFECTION an infection that is time limited.

ADDRESSOGRAPH MACHINE a device used to imprint client information contained on the hospital card onto client documents.

AEROBIC BACTERIA bacteria that require oxygen to grow.

AFFINITY SCHEDULING (ALSO CALLED CLUSTER, CATEGORIZATION, OR ANALOGOUS SCHEDULING) scheduling similar appointments together, for example, scheduling physical examinations on a certain day.

ALLIED HEALTH CARE any duty or profession that supports primary healthcare professionals, such as physicians, in delivering health-care services.

ALTERNATIVE HEALTH CARE OR COMPLEMENTARY HEALTH CARE nontraditional methods and practices, based on a natural approach, including chiropractic, acupuncture, massage, and aromatherapy.

ANABOLISM assimilating nutrients and building up the complex molecules of living tissue.

ANAEROBIC BACTERIA bacteria that do not require oxygen to grow.

ANGIOCATHETER OR ANGIOCATH a plastic tube, usually attached to the puncturing needle, inserted into a blood vessel for infusion, injection, or pressure monitoring.

ANTENATAL before birth.

ANTIBODY a protein specific to a certain antigen which weakens or destroys pathogens.

ANTIGEN—ANTIBODY RESPONSE the process by which the immune system produces special substances to fight off foreign substances

ANTIGEN a pathogen or any other substance that induces an antibody response.

ANTISEPSIS the process of reducing microorganisms to prevent the spread of infection.

ANTISEPTIC a cleansing agent that can be applied to living tissue to destroy pathogens.

APICAL PULSE measurement of the heartbeat near the heart, usually using a stethoscope.

ARCHIVE to remove a file from active status and store it in a secondary location or on a secondary medium.

ARRHYTHMIA loss of normal rhythm of the heartbeat.

ARTERIES vessels that carry blood away from the heart.

ARTERIOLES small branches of arteries.

ARTERIOSCLEROSIS hardening of the arteries; reduces blood flow.

ASEPSIS a state in which pathogens are absent or reduced. There are two principal types of asepsis: medical and surgical.

ASTHMA a disease that affects the air passages in the lung, causing wheezing and shortness of breath.

ASYMPTOMATIC without clinical signs or symptoms.

ATHEROSCLEROSIS arteriosclerosis due to deposits of fat in arterial walls.

ATRIAL FIBRILLATION an abnormality of heart rhythm in which chambers of the heart no longer beat in synchrony, with the atrium beating much faster than the ventricles. The heart rate is fast and irregular.

ATTENUATED ORGANISM one that has been weakened for use in a vaccine. It cannot produce the disease, but will stimulate the body to produce antibodies.

ATTRIBUTE an inborn personal quality or characteristic.

AUSCULTATE listen to the sounds made by a body structure as a diagnostic method.

AUTOCLAVE a device using steam for sterilization.

AUTOPSY the examination of a body to determine the cause of death and/or to identify disease processes.

AUXILIARY FILE a temporary filing space for files in current use.

BACTERICIDAL killing microorganisms.

BACTERIOSTATIC reducing or inhibiting the number of microorganisms.

BARD BUTTON (MIC DEVICE) a feeding device placed permanently in the stomach to facilitate supplemental feedings.

BEHAVIOUR a person's discernible responses and actions.

BENEFICIARY a person eligible to receive insurance benefits under specified conditions.

BENEFICIARY a person eligible to receive insurance benefits under specified conditions.

BILLING CODE, SERVICE CODE, OR ITEM CODE a number that identifies the service a provider has performed for an insured client and that determines the fee to be paid by a provincial or territorial health plan.

BOLUS the usually rapid infusion of additional IV fluids or an IV, IM, or S/C medication in addition to the base amount ordered for the client.

BOWEL OBSTRUCTION a blockage in the intestines that prevents their contents from moving forward.

BOWEL RESECTION (ANASTOMOSIS OR END-TO-END ANASTOMOSIS) surgery wherein a section of bowel is removed, and the remaining bowel is reconnected.

BOWEL SOUNDS PRESENT (BSP) the audible return of gastrointestinal movement or function, also called peristalsis.

BRADYCARDIA extremely slow heartbeat.

BRUIT a sound, especially an abnormal one, heard on auscultation or by ultrasound.

CANNULA an inner tube.

CAPILLARIES thin, minute blood vessels joining the arterioles and venules, through which oxygen transfer occurs.

CAPITATION (POPULATION-BASED FUNDING) a funding system that pays a physician a given amount per patient enrolled, regardless of the number of services performed.

CARCINOGENICITY the ability of a substance to cause cancer.

CATABOLISM breaking down complex chemical compounds in nutrients into simpler ones, releasing energy used as fuel by the body.

CC cubic centimetre; 1 cc equals 1 millilitre (1 mL). In hospitals, cc is used more often than mL.

CEREBRAL VASCULAR ACCIDENT (CVA) OR STROKE damage to the brain that occurs when the blood supply to an area of the brain is diminished or occluded completely.

CHRONIC CARE care for someone with a chronic illness, that is, one that typically progresses slowly but lasts for a long time, often lifelong.

CHRONIC INFECTION one that is persistent over a long period, perhaps for life.

CHRONIC OBSTRUCTIVE LUNG DISEASE (COLD) OR CHRONIC OBSTRUCTIVE PULMONARY DISEASE (COPD) any chronic lung condition in which the flow of expired air is slowed down.

CIRCUMORAL PALLOR a pale area around the mouth.

CLAPPING OR PERCUSSION using cupped hands to gently but firmly strike affected regions of the chest to move secretions.

CLIENT a person seeking or receiving health care; synonymous with patient, but suggests a more active role.

CLINIC a facility providing medical care on an outpatient basis. Many clinics have a specialty, such as ongoing care for diabetes or cancer.

CLINICAL SECRETARY (SC) OR WARD CLERK a health office professional working in a hospital; an individual who assumes responsibilities for the secretarial, clerical, communication, and other designated needs of a hospital unit or department.

COLLABORATIVE PARTNERSHIP the relationship among hospitals that have entered into an agreement to form a partnership, sharing clinical and administrative responsibilities.

COLOSTOMY a surgical procedure that creates an artificial opening from the colon to the surface of the abdomen, through which feces are excreted.

COMBINATION SCHEDULING OR BLENDED SCHEDULING a combination of affinity and random scheduling.

COMPUTED TOMOGRAPHY (CT) a type of X-ray that produces three-dimensional images of cross-sections of body parts.

CONGESTIVE HEART FAILURE (CHF) a condition in which a weakened heart is unable to pump all of the blood out of the lungs each time it beats. Blood pools at the bottom of the lungs, interfering with breathing.

CONTAGIOUS OR COMMUNICABLE DISEASE a disease that is spread from person to person.

CONTAMINATION the presence of pathogens on an object.

CONTROLLED DRUGS drugs defined by federal law to which special rules apply because they are liable to be abused.

CORE (INTERNAL) TEMPERATURE the temperature of vital organs, such as the brain, heart, and liver.

CORE COMPETENCY the basic or essential skills that one needs to succeed in a particular profession.

COUPLING two heartbeats close together, followed by a space.

CRACKLES OR CREPITATION sounds produced by air passing over airway secretions.

CRASH CART a cart carrying the supplies needed for immediate treatment of a heart attack.

CREDENTIALLING a process whereby a peer group judges an individual's qualifications to perform certain services.

CRITICAL VALUE a test result that so deviates from normal that it causes concern for the client's immediate well-being.

CRITICAL VALUE one that indicates a life-threatening situation and requires immediate attention.

CRITICALLY ILL experiencing life-threatening problems; in medical crisis.

CROSS-COVERAGE moving from one area to another, or covering two units.

CULTURE the languages, beliefs, values, norms, behaviours, and even material objects that are passed from one generation to the next.

CYANOSIS blue or purplish tinge to skin, mucous membranes, or nailbeds.

CYSTECTOMY surgical removal of the urinary bladder.

CYSTOSCOPE a long thin flexible instrument with a light at the end used to examine the bladder. It is inserted through the urethra and threaded up into the bladder.

DAY SURGERY surgery conducted with a hospital stay of less than 24 hours.

DEDUCTIBLE the portion of a benefit that a beneficiary must pay before receiving coverage.

DEEP SUCTIONING introducing the suction catheter into the lower trachea and bronchi.

DEREGULATED (of a service) removed from a province's or territory's fee schedule so that it is no longer insured under that jurisdiction's health plan.

DIASTOLIC PRESSURE the pressure of the vascular walls when the hear is relaxing.

DISCHARGE any release from a health-care facility by doctor's orders.

DISINFECTANT a chemical substance that destroys or eliminates specific species of infectious microorganisms. It is not usually effective against bacterial spores.

DISINFECTION a more thorough removal of contaminants than sanitization but less thorough than sterilization.

DISTAL the part farthest from the body.

DISTRIBUTION the process by which metabolites are transported to various parts of the body.

DIVERTICULITIS inflammation of a sac-like bulge that may develop in the wall of the large intestine.

DOCTORS' ORDERS written or oral directions given by a physician to the nursing staff and other health professionals regarding the care, medications, treatment, and laboratory and diagnostic tests a client is to receive while in hospital.

DOUBLE BOOKING OR DOUBLE-COLUMN BOOKING booking two client appointments at the same time, on the assumption that one of the appointments will involve little of the doctor's time.

DRESSING TRAY a specially prepared sterile tray containing the basic equipment to change a dressing on a wound or surgical incision. It contains a K-basin, 4 × 4 gauze dressings, a galley cup (a small metal or glass cup about the size of a shot glass used for cleansing solutions), and usually two sets of disposable forceps.

DROPS PER MINUTE (GTT/MIN) a measure of the rate of IV infusion.

DYSPHAGIA difficulty swallowing.

DYSPNEA shortness of breath; a subjective difficulty or distress in breathing.

ELECTIVE SURGERY nonemergency, planned surgery, booked in advance.

ELECTIVE SURGERY surgery that is necessary but not an emergency and can therefore be booked in advance. Examples of elective surgery include removal of a tumour, a hip replacement, or a hysterectomy. Appendicitis usually necessitates emergency surgery.

ELECTRONIC DATA TRANSFER (EDT) vehicle for the electronic transmission of medical claims from the source computer to the Ministry's mainframe computer.

ELECTRONIC DATA TRANSFER exchanging information electronically between computers in a process similar to e-mail; a common method of claims submission.

EMBOLISM obstruction of a blood vessel by a blood clot, an air bubble, or foreign matter.

EMERGENTOLOGIST a physician specializing in emergency medicine.

EMESIS BASIN (KIDNEY BASIN OR K-BASIN) a small basin, usually kidney shaped, used for clients to vomit into or cough up sputum or phlegm. They are also used to hold solutions for a variety of purposes. They may be ordered sterile or just clean.

EMPHYSEMA a disease characterized by gradual destruction of the alveoli, which fuse to form larger air spaces. Exchange of oxygen and carbon dioxide through these larger air sacs is inadequate.

ENDOSCOPY examination of a canal, such as the colon, with an endoscope: a thin tube with lenses to allow visualization.

ENDOTRACHEAL SUCTIONING suctioning through an artificial airway known as a tracheostomy.

ENEMA the introduction of liquid into the rectum through the anus for cleansing the bowel and for stimulating evacuation of the bowels.

ENTERAL FEED feeding by tube directly into the gastrointestinal system.

ENZYME a protein capable of initiating a chemical reaction that involves the formation or breakage of chemical bonds. When muscle damage or death occurs, enzymes within the muscle cell are released into the circulating blood.

EPISIOTOMY a surgical incision made into the perineum to facilitate the vaginal delivery of a baby.

ETHNIC relating to groups of people with a common racial, religious, linguistic, or cultural heritage.

ETHNOCENTRISM the tendency to use our own culture's standards as the yardstick to judge everyone; the belief in the superiority of our own group or culture.

EXACERBATION a period in which a chronic infection shows symptoms.

EXACERBATION the phase of a chronic disease characterized by a return of clinical signs or symptoms.

EXTERNSHIP a cooperative or workplace experience or period of training for a student that is provided by the student's educational facility.

EXTRA BILLING charging a client more than the amount paid by the provincial/territorial health plan for a medically necessary service.

FAMILY HEALTH NETWORK (ALSO KNOWN AS PRIMARY CARE NETWORK OR FAMILY CARE NETWORK) a group of physicians operating in accordance with the policies and principles set out by the primary care reform initiative in their province or territory.

FAMILY PHYSICIAN an MD with a specialty in family medicine who looks after the general medical needs of a varied practice population.

FEBRILE involving fever.

FEE FOR SERVICE a system under which a provider is paid for each insured service rendered to an insured client.

FIXED OILS (also called base or carrier oils) oils, extracted primarily from plants, that do not evaporate.

FLAG (of a chart) to draw attention to a new entry by sticking a coloured marker in, placing a coloured sticker on the back, or using some other device to visually draw attention.

FLATUS gas that is passed rectally.

FLUID RETENTION an accumulation of fluid in body tissues or body cavities.

FUNDUS the top of the uterus. Measuring how high the fundus is in the abdomen provides valuable information about the size of the uterus and the progression of fetal growth.

GASTRIC SUCTION gentle suction applied to a tube placed in the stomach to remove excessive secretions, such as saliva and gastric juices, that tend to accumulate in the stomach after surgery or trauma because the intestine is sluggish. This can prevent or relieve nausea and vomiting.

GASTRITIS inflammation of the stomach.

GASTROSTOMY TUBE (G-TUBE) a feeding tube inserted through an incision in the abdomen into the stomach.

GLOBAL BUDGET any arrangement in which a facility or provider receives a fixed amount of money for medical services, regardless of patient volume, length of stay, or services rendered.

HEAD INJURY ROUTINE a special assessment for a client who has had head trauma or surgery, including checks on neurological functioning such as verbal response and pupil dilation.

HEALTH OFFICE PROFESSIONAL (HOP) a graduate from an accredited health office administration program who assumes administrative, communication, and/or clinical responsibilities in a health-care setting. Depending on the occupational setting, this graduate may be assigned such job titles as medical secretary, medical office assistant,